W9-CSN-732

WASHING "THE GREAT UNWASHED"

# Washing
# "The Great Unwashed"

## Public Baths in
## Urban America,
## 1840-1920

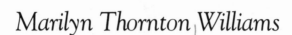

*Marilyn Thornton Williams*

Ohio State University Press

*Columbus*

Library of Congress Cataloging-in-Publication Data

Williams, Marilyn T.
Washing "the great unwashed" : public baths in urban America,
1840-1920 / Marilyn Thornton Williams.
p.    cm.—(Urban life and urban landscape series)
Includes bibliography (p.    ) and index.
ISBN 0-8142-0537-2
1. Baths, Public—United States—19th century—History.    2. Baths,
Public—United States—20th century—History.    I. Title.
II. Series.
RA605.W54    1991
613'.41'0973—dc20        90-14212
CIP

⊗ The paper in this book meets the guidelines for permanence and
durability of the Committee on Production Guidelines for Book
Longevity of the Council on Library Resources.

Printed in the U.S.A.

9   8   7   6   5   4   3   2   1

*To my mother*
LYDIA MARCOTTE THORNTON
*and to the memory of my father*
WILLIAM E. THORNTON

The "great unwashed" were not so from choice.

—JACOB A. RIIS

# Contents

# Illustrations

## Plates

## Tables

## Illustrations

**Maps**

# Acknowledgments

It is a pleasure after so many years to be able to express my gratitude to the many people and organizations who made this project possible, although words seem inadequate to the task.

My first thanks go to Bayrd Still, an ideal mentor and friend, who nurtured this project from its beginnings as a seminar paper through its appearance as a dissertation. His kind and thoughtful guidance has been invaluable.

I am very obliged to the many friends and colleagues who have read portions of this book and offered excellent suggestions and astute criticisms. Thanks to the members of the Reading Group on Cities: Cathy Alexander, Jane Allen, Natalie Auerbach, Selma Berrol, Barbara Blumberg, Betty Boyd Caroli, Kathleen Centola, Joyce Gold, Nora Mandel, Jean Mensch, and Carol Nuels-Bates. I am especially indebted to my dear friend Barbara J. Harris, who gave me understanding, encouragement, and inspiration as well as sound editorial advice.

I also wish to thank the members of the Columbia University Seminar on the City for their comments on an early version of the New York City chapter and Jack Tager for his comments on a version of the Boston chapter.

Without the assistance of many libraries, this book would not have been possible. My gratitude to the staffs of the Pace University Library, the New York Public Library, the New York University Library, the Library of Congress, the Rare Book and Manuscript Library, Columbia University, the Library of the New York Academy of Medicine, and the Library of the Historical Society of Pennsylvania.

I am grateful to the many members of the Pace University community who contributed to the completion of this book. My thanks to Dean Joseph Houle and Provost Joseph Pastore for their interest and support, as well as for financial assistance for the preparation of maps and photographs. A sabbatical and summer research grants gave me time to complete revisions, and a grant from the Scholarly Research Committee covered typing costs for the first draft. My colleagues Jean Fagan Yellin and Joan Roland were always interested and encouraging. The Word Processing Department under Blanche Amelkin and Jackie Myers produced the tables and appendixes. I offer special thanks to Michael Galama, who drew the maps and the floor plans. Over the years my students have asked the right questions and enabled me to think through many historical issues.

For their many thoughtful and helpful suggestions, I am indebted to the editors of this series, Henry D. Shapiro and Zane L. Miller. I also appreciate the assistance of Alex Holzman and Charlotte Dihoff of Ohio State University Press.

Earlier versions of portions of this book have been published in the *Maryland Historical Magazine* 77 (Spring 1977), 118–31; *Journal of Urban History* 7 (November, 1980), 49–81; and in Jack Tager and John W. Ifkovic, eds., *Massachusetts in the Gilded Age: Selected Essays* (Amherst: University of Massachusetts Press, 1985). My thanks to these publishers for permission to reprint in this work.

Finally, my gratitude to the members of my family for their confidence in me, to Roger for timely research assistance, to Karen for help with photographs, and to Jocelyn and Karen, for feminist solidarity, humor, and perspective.

# Introduction

Deny to the poor those advantages which are possessed by the rich
and you intensify discontent. When the poor are so very poor as
they are in our cities and have neither the knowledge nor customs
nor initiative to be other than as they are, it is a duty of the public,
as its own government, to educate them out of their condition, to
give baths to them that they may be fit to associate together and
with others without offense and without danger. A man cannot
truly respect himself who is dirty. Stimulate the habit of cleanliness
and we increase the safety of our cities. And give over the idea that a
free bath is any more of a "gratuity" than the right to walk in the
public streets.

—*BROOKLYN DAILY EAGLE*, SEPT. 12, 1897

By 1897, when a New York City newspaper editor wrote these words,
public baths were accepted as one of the important services which progressive American cities must provide for their poorer citizens. Personal
cleanliness had become a necessity, not only for social acceptability and
public health but also as a symbol of middle-class status, good character,
self-respect, and membership in the civic community. If slum tenements
failed to provide the poor with bathing facilities so that they could attain
the proper standards of cleanliness, then cities must provide public baths
to wash the great unwashed. Cleanliness had become a right of all citizens.

Bath reformers used the generic term "public bath" to refer to a bathhouse built, either by a municipality or a charitable organization or an
individual, specifically to serve the poor (they were either free or charged
a small fee). Municipal baths were those built by city governments, but
these baths were usually called public baths and this practice has been
followed in this book. Private bathhouses, which were found in most

nineteenth-century cities, were commercial enterprises that also were open to the public but generally were too expensive for the poorer classes.

This book is a study of the history of the public bath movement, an almost forgotten urban reform. Public baths were one of the many solutions proposed by nineteenth-century American reformers when they were faced with the numerous social problems presented by unprecedented urban growth and congested slums. The demands that cities furnish public baths for their poorer citizens began in the 1840s, continued through the ensuing decades, and culminated during the Progessive Era, when many American cities constructed public baths in slum neighborhoods. Although the public bath movement justifiably may be seen as part of the massive urban social reform of the Progressive Era, the arguments put forward by the bath reformers in that era echo those of earlier advocates and were based on previous experiences. In one case even their actions were the same. In 1851 the New York Association for Improving the Condition of the Poor erected a public bath on New York City's Lower East Side but closed it ten years later because it was not self-supporting; forty years later it built another public bath in the same area that was successful and became a prototype for future public baths.

From the beginning the demand for public baths was part of the wider demand for public health reform. Bath reformers maintained that baths would safeguard the health, not only of the poor but of all people in the city. But cleanliness would do more for the poor; bath advocates maintained that it would improve their moral character and make them better citizens. In fact as personal cleanliness became a hallmark of American middle-class status and respectability, it made the separation between the classes wider. Public baths would help bridge this gap, bath reformers maintained, and thus achieve one small measure of social justice.

The movement for public baths was also part of the effort to improve the urban environment and can be compared to movements for public parks, playgrounds, tenement house reform, and effective garbage collection. All these improvements would make the lives of city dwellers, especially the poor, healthier and more pleasant.

The history of the public bath movement illustrates the changing conceptions of the duties and functions of urban governments and the trend toward constantly expanding responsibilities. Antebellum cities did not seriously consider the demands for public baths; Gilded Age cities built floating baths on their riverfronts and beach baths on their waterfronts but did not build the more expensive year-round baths. Progressive Era cities built public baths; some of them built very complete bath systems. New York City, for example, built twenty-five public baths and spent approximately four million early twentieth-century dollars in the effort.

The first demands for public baths came in the midst of the massive waves of Irish immigration, and the movement achieved its greatest success during the greater waves of eastern and southern European immigration at the turn of the century. Bath reformers asserted that public baths would assist in Americanizing the immigrants, and it appears that this group concerned them the most because the majority of public baths were located in immigrant neighborhoods.

The organization of this book proceeds from the general to the specific. Beginning with a brief history of public baths, chapter 1 surveys the development of the American obsession with personal cleanliness. In the mid-nineteenth century, many factors—including economic depression, the burgeoning urban slums of Irish immigrants, the water cure craze and other health reforms which connected cleanliness to health, the threat of epidemics, and the existing bath systems of large European cities—all contributed to the growing demand for public baths. The provision of water and sewage systems in large cities as well as technological developments, such as bathtubs with attached plumbing, gave the private bath first to the affluent and then to the middle class and made public baths for the poor feasible.

Chapter 2 traces the growing demand for public baths in the Progressive Era as new waves of southern and eastern European immigrants and increasing acceptance of the germ theory of disease in the 1880s added new impetus to the cause. Bath reformers grew more numerous, their arguments became more sophisticated and their demands more insistent. In this era of great urban reform the public bath movement reached its peak and achieved success.

Chapters 3–5 explore how and why this reform was achieved in five American cities: New York, Boston, Chicago, Philadelphia, and Baltimore. These cities were chosen as case studies for several reasons. Excluding St. Louis, they were the largest cities in the country in 1900.[1] Their bath reformers were the most active and successful, and these cities had the most extensive and well-publicized bath systems. Their municipal governments responded to demands for public baths in different ways and produced very different results or did not respond at all and left the building of baths to private philanthropy.

The study of the bath movement in these cities illuminates many of the issues surrounding progressive social reform and reveals the interplay between reformers and city governments. It identifies and explores the common interests of the issue-focused public bath reformers and their supporters and considers the question of the participation of the poor, for whom the baths were intended. The reactions of municipal governments and their leaders, both political bosses and reform mayors, were varied. Why did some cities build bath systems for their poorer citizens and others leave the task to private philanthropy? The discourse of the movement reveals the mixed motives and messages of those interested in urban reform in this period. Their goals and their rhetoric did not always conform to the actual results that they achieved. The comparative importance of social justice, social control, and public health in the motives of the bath reformers illustrates the complexity of urban reform in this era.

At the peak of its success the bath movement was organized both nationally and internationally. The activities of the American Association for Promoting Hygiene and Public Baths are discussed in chapter 6.

Finally, chapter 7 assesses the success, meaning, and lasting legacy of the public bath movement. In preaching the gospel of cleanliness, the public bath reformers wished to extend to the great unwashed in large American cities one of the amenities that their more affluent neighbors enjoyed and, in so doing, hoped to improve the lives of all the citizens of urban communities.

# 1

## Origins of the Public Bath
## Movement, 1840–1890

The advance of civilization is largely measured by the victories of
mankind over its greatest enemy—dirt.

—JOSIAH QUINCY

In his influential book *How the Other Half Lives,* journalist and social reformer Jacob A. Riis wrote about the children of Jewish immigrants on
New York City's Lower East Side:

The majority of the children seek the public school, where they are received
sometimes with some misgivings on the part of the teachers, who find it necessary to inculcate lessons of cleanliness in the worst cases by practical demonstra-
tions with soap and water. "He took the soap as if it were some animal," said one
of these teachers to me after such an experiment upon a new pupil, "and wiped
three fingers across his face. He called that washing."

To correct this situation, every day the teachers asked the children,
"What must I do to be healthy?" and the children responded:

I must keep my skin clean
Wear clean clothes
Breathe pure air
And live in the sunlight

Difficult as it may have been for these immigrant children living in New
York City's tenements to follow the rules they recited, they were learning
officially that personal cleanliness was very important in America.[1]

By 1890, when Riis' book was published, most Americans had come to
believe, as we do today, that the desire to be clean was almost innate and

that to go without bathing for any length of time voluntarily was inconceivable and repugnant. This cultural norm developed gradually during the nineteenth century at the same time that city growth, immigration, and developing urban slums prevented the urban poor from conforming to the accepted standard of cleanliness.

For those Americans interested in improving the lot of the poor, the solution to their lack of personal cleanliness was the public bath which would be open year-round. The demand for public baths initially appeared in the 1840s in response to a variety of factors. The widespread urban suffering among the poor caused by the Panic of 1837 and its aftermath, the massive emigration from Ireland, and mushrooming urban growth presented Americans with new and seemingly insurmountable problems. New York City's population had increased from 202,598 in 1830 to 515,547 in 1850, Philadelphia's from 161,410 to 340,045, and Boston's from 61,392 to 136,881. Most of the 1.2 million Irish immigrants fleeing the famine between 1845 and 1854 got no farther than these port cities, where they lived in districts filled with unimaginable filth and squalor. To Americans these burgeoning slums with their poverty, vice, crime, disorder, drunkenness, and apparently unassimilable immigrants were a threat to the social fabric of American society. Throughout the nineteenth century several generations of urban reformers grappled with the intractable problems generated by the slums, proposed various solutions, found them wanting, and tried new ones.[2]

However, the problem of the cleanliness of slum dwellers and the solution proposed—public baths—were constant from the 1840s through the Progressive Era. Although urban slums initially generated this concern, a number of other factors contributed to the rising interest in the cleanliness of the poor.

## The European Influence

Historical precedent and the European experience were very influential in stimulating the interest of American public bath reformers. These leaders harked back to classical antiquity and often referred to the lavish public baths of the Romans and to the religiously connected bathing of the ancient Hebrews and Egyptians. With the fall of Rome, however, public baths declined in western Europe and did not reappear again until the period of the Crusades. The contact between the Crusaders and the

Byzantine and Moslem empires apparently revived the institution of the public bath. From the thirteenth to the seventeenth centuries public baths equipped with small communal bathing pools and steam baths could usually be found in the cities and larger towns of Europe and were licensed by the municipalities. These bathhouses also were often places of amusement which furnished food, drink, music, and women and thus were sometimes the subject of intense antibath campaigns by the clergy. In the fifteenth century separate bathhouses for men and women became the vogue. In the sixteenth century, when syphilis became a new health problem, these medieval communal baths were seen as a focus of infection and fell into disfavor. The influence of the Reformation and Counter-Reformation also played a role as these bathhouses were perceived as places of nakedness, immorality, and sin. By the end of the seventeenth century public baths had vanished from the urban scene in western Europe.[3]

With the disappearance of the medieval public bath, complete, all-over bathing went out of fashion. Private homes lacked baths and for a time bathing was considered dangerous to the health. By the late seventeenth century, however, interest in bathing revived, as indicated by the one hundred bathrooms Louis XIV built at Versailles, but waned when they were dismantled during the eighteenth century. Toward the middle of the eighteenth century, however, a vogue for bathing in the summer arose and commercial public baths began to appear. This revival of interest in bathing focused especially on medicinal baths. The development of the city of Bath, England, at this time publicized the idea of public establishments for bathing.[4]

The industrial revolution, expanding urban populations, the growth of urban slums, a series of cholera epidemics beginning in the 1830s, and rising middle-class standards of personal cleanliness all combined to give impetus to the municipal bath movement in Europe, as they did later for the one in America. The movement began in England in the 1820s, reached a peak in the 1840s, and spread to the Continent in the second half of the nineteenth century.[5]

In England the first indoor public bath built for the people at public expense was the St. George's Bath in Liverpool, opened in 1828. Fees were charged although the bath had been built with public funds. This bath included two large swimming pools, two small plunge baths (smaller pools), eleven private tub baths, one vapor (steam) bath, and one shower bath. In 1842 the Frederick Street Baths and Washhouse opened in the same city. This was the first bath in England to include a public washhouse (laundry) as well as bath facilities, which eventually became the norm for all baths in that country. In 1844 the philanthropic London Association for Promoting Cleanliness Among the Poor built a bath-house and laundry in East Smithfield. But the English municipal bath movement achieved its greatest success with the passage of "An Act to Encourage the Establishment of Public Baths and Washhouses" in 1846, a law probably passed partly because of increasing Irish immigration to English cities, especially Liverpool, and fear of cholera.[6]

This enabling legislation, which was voluntary rather than compul-sory, provided that any local government could build and maintain pub-lic baths and washhouses at public expense to be administered by a board of commissioners. The baths could furnish both first- and second-class accommodations (later amended to include third-class) in swim-ming pools, warm and cold tub baths, vapor baths, warm and cold shower baths, and public laundries. The legislation called for a minimum of twice as many baths for the laboring classes (second or third class) as for the upper classes (first or second class). The baths were not to be free and a minimum fee of one pence (later two pence) was established for a second-class cold bath.[7]

By 1896 more than 200 municipalities in the British Isles were main-taining public baths. The average English municipal bath was large, handsome, and costly. For example, the Hornsey Road Baths, erected in 1892 by the Parish of St. Mary's, Islington, London, cost $175,194. For men it had a first-class swimming pool of 32 by 100 feet with 71 dressing rooms, and for women a swimming pool measuring 25 by 75 feet; also furnished were 108 private tub and shower baths, lavatories, and a public laundry with accommodation for 40 washers. Such baths often included a large meeting or lecture hall, kitchen, and refreshment rooms as well as a steam bath.[8]

These English baths were extensively patronized by the middle class, who, unlike their American counterparts, lacked bath facilities in their homes, but the baths were often criticized as being too imposing and expensive for the working class. Some suggested a separate entrance for the poor or a reduction of the fee to one pence. Others suggested the building of "cottage baths," simpler, smaller, and cheaper baths to be located in slum districts. Apparently very few cottage baths were ever built. In the United States, also, the elaborateness of the public baths, especially those built in New York City, was often attacked.[9]

Whereas large and elaborate baths were most popular in England, more variation was found in continental Europe. In France, for example, bath facilities were less important than public laundries, although after permissive legislation was passed in 1851 most major French cities had a public bathhouse.[10]

Germany and Austria had a wide variety of municipal bathing establishments. Although laundries were rarely part of German and Austrian bath systems, they did include large elaborate bathing facilities like those in England and were an important source of civic pride. The magnificent Stuttgart Bathhouse, for example, contained 2 swimming pools, 1 for men and 1 for women, 300 dressing rooms, 102 tub baths, 2 Russian-Roman baths for men and women, 2 cold water cure sections for men and women, a sun bath, and a bath for dogs. Its patrons were largely from the middle class, who, like their English counterparts, lacked bathing facilities in their homes. In 1883, however, Dr. Oscar Lasser of the University of Berlin set up his model "People's Bath" at the Berlin Hygiene Exhibition. This bath was a small corrugated-iron structure divided into ten cubicles, five for men and five for women, each equipped with a shower. At the exhibition several thousand visitors enjoyed a hot water shower at ten pfennigs each, thus proving that it was technologically feasible and inexpensive to use showers in public bath facilities. Following this example, most German and Austrian municipalities, beginning with Vienna in 1887, in addition to their large baths operated a number of small and modest Volksbad for the lower classes, with between 10 and 80 warm and cold showers. In Germany, school shower baths and workers' shower baths (located at factories) were also common.[11]

The first use of the shower or rain bath for mass bathing was credited to either the French or the German military, who set up showers in soldiers' barracks in the middle 1800s. Shower baths rather than tub baths became the ideal type of public bath according to the public bath advocates. Showers were less expensive to build, easier to keep clean and sanitary, used less water, and took less time than tub baths when large numbers of people had to be accommodated.[12]

By 1891 smaller numbers of municipal baths could also be found in most European countries, including Belgium, Holland, Italy, Hungary, Norway, and Sweden. Buenos Aires had the only municipal bath in

South America. Although most of these foreign municipal baths were very inexpensive for patrons, apparently none of them was free.[13]

The extent and success of European municipal bath systems were key elements in the arguments of American bath advocates. Cultural deference as well as emulation played a role. Not only was the United States shown to be lagging behind Europe in this respect, but the European experience had proven that the operation of such systems was feasible. As the Boston bath proponent Edward M. Hartwell wrote, "The teaching of European experience . . . can hardly fail to prove helpful and instructive to those who are endeavoring to ameliorate the conditions due to urban crowding in the United States." American bath proponents also occasionally referred to the Japanese system of public baths as an example of that nation's intelligence and progressiveness.[14]

## American Origins

Although American public bath advocates were inspired by the imposing municipal baths of European cities and considered them to be one of the important amenities which cities should provide for their citizens, American public baths were built for the poor. Like their European counterparts, middle-class Americans during the nineteenth century had become convinced of the necessity for bodily cleanliness but built bathrooms in their homes rather than public baths.

In the colonial period Americans followed the European custom of seldom bathing the entire body. By the middle of the eighteenth century, however, the vogue for spas, mineral springs, and watering places had crossed the Atlantic. There was some resistance to the development of spring baths on the grounds of immorality. For example, in 1761, when plans were made to develop the chalybeate spring in the Northern Liberties area of Philadelphia, the Protestant ministers petitioned the governor to prevent a lottery to be held for the purpose of "erecting public Gardens with Baths and Bagnios among us. Were a Hot and Cold Bath necessary to the Health of the Inhabitants of the City," they contended, "they might at a small expense be added to the Hospital." They insisted that a stop must be put to the people's "Immoderate and Growing Fondness for Pleasure, Luxury, Gaming, Dissipation, and their concommittant Vices." But this kind of disapproval failed to moderate what became a rage for bathing in and drinking natural spring or mineral waters as a form of medical treatment or at least as a general aid to good health.[15]

In the 1760s and 1770s numerous baths and watering places appeared where nature had provided springs or mineral waters. One of the most popular of these spas was at Stafford Springs, Connecticut, which had the reputation of curing diseases such as gout, sterility, rheumatism, and hysteria. Feeling in ill health, John Adams spent four days there in 1771. He recorded in his *Diary:* "I drank plentifully of the water; it had the taste of fair water with an infusion of steel. . . . I plunged in twice, but the second time was superfluous and did me more hurt than good; it is very cold indeed." He later noted somewhat skeptically, "The journey was of use to me whether the waters were or not." The most renowned and fashionable southern watering place was Berkeley Warm Springs, Virginia, where the social elite of the southern colonies gathered. George Washington took the water there on three occasions, one of which was a vain attempt to cure his stepdaughter, Patsy Custis, of her epilepsy. Philip Fithian also visited this spa and noted the very active social life of the patrons, who enjoyed cardplaying and balls as well as the baths.[16]

As Americans became accustomed to bathing at natural springs, they also apparently wished to be able to bathe closer to home, for commercially operated public bathhouses began to appear in American cities in the last decades of the eighteenth century. In 1792 Nicholas Denise of New York City announced that he had "just established though at great expense . . . a very convenient Bathing House, having eight rooms, in every one of which Baths may be had with either fresh, salt or warm water. . . . The said place is at his home called Bellevue on the East River; prices fixed at 4s per person and attendance at the house at any time." Often these commercial public baths advertised that in addition to bathing facilities, they maintained a garden, teahouse, or restaurant for the enjoyment of their patrons. At this point all-over bathing was considered a form of recreation and diversion but not a necessity. Many of these baths were open only in the summer months.[17]

Before the Civil War, as municipal water systems were constructed and produced plentiful and cheap water, commercial bathhouses became a fairly common fixture in American cities. They offered to their middle- and upper-class patrons a variety of baths: Russian (similar to sauna baths), steam, vapor, mud, or swimming, as well as other amenities. The new western cities kept pace with their eastern counterparts. By the

1840s Chicago, for example, could boast three bathhouses, one with a section for women.[18]

At the same time that commercial public baths became commonplace, well-to-do Americans began to acquire bathing facilities in their homes. Elizabeth Drinker recorded in her diary in 1798 the installation of a shower bath in the backyard of her Philadelphia townhouse. A year later she described her experience as she finally "went into the Shower bath. I bore it better than I expected, not having been wett all over at once, for 28 years past." Here she was alluding to the fact that her last complete bath had been in 1771, when she had bathed in the mineral springs at Bristol, New Jersey. Concurrently, "bathing tubs" made of wood and lined with tin became available, and the Drinkers bought one of these in 1803. Owing to the trouble of filling the tub, however, the male Drinkers continued to patronize the public baths sporadically.[19]

The establishment of municipal water systems which brought running water into the homes of the middle and upper classes and the construction of sewage systems which removed it, as well as the invention of bathtubs with attached plumbing and water heaters, simplified bathing at home. When George Templeton Strong of New York City acquired such facilities in 1843 he wrote enthusiastically in his *Diary*, "Tried our new bath room last night for the first time and propose to repeat the experiment this evening. It's a great luxury—worth the cost of the whole building." Two weeks later he noted, "I've led rather an amphibious life for the last week, paddling in the bathing tub every night and constantly making new discoveries in the art and mystery of ablution. Taking a shower bath upside down is the last novelty." Although very few Americans of any social class bathed as frequently as Strong, more and more had the facilities to do so. It was not until 1851, however, that Millard Fillmore had a bathtub installed in the White House amid complaints about unnecessary expense.[20]

Further impetus to the custom of bathing by getting "wett all over at once" came from the water cure craze of the 1840s and 1850s, which reinforced the association between bathing and health. Developed by Vincent Priessnitz in Silesia, the water cure, or hydropathy, became extremely popular in the United States as a treatment for almost all ailments. Based on the concept that water was the sustainer of life, treatments consisted of a variety of baths, wet compresses, steam, water massage, copious drinking of cold water, exercise, and a simple diet. Between the 1840s and 1880s over 200 water cure centers were established throughout the United States with women as their chief clientele. The *Water Cure Journal*, with "Wash and Be Healed" as its motto, had a wide readership.[21]

Influenced by the message of hydropathy, other health reformers of the mid-nineteenth century also urged frequent bathing. Sylvester Graham's regimen included taking a bath "in very warm water at least three times a week." Catherine Beecher, who had personally benefited from the water cure, denounced those Americans who washed only "the face, feet, hands and neck" and proclaimed that "it is a rule of health that the whole body should be washed every day." Although the water cure craze subsided by the time of the Civil War, hydrotherapy, as it came to be called, persisted as a treatment for some diseases, and bathing was seen as necessary for good health. Simon Baruch, an orthodox physician and a national leader of the public bath movement (and Bernard Baruch's father), was a leading proponent of hydrotherapy.[22]

American interest in health reform and physical fitness, however, did not subside as vogues for various diets, exercise regimens, and sports flourished and declined throughout the nineteenth century to the present day. Health reformers remained almost unanimous in affirming the importance of personal cleanliness and regular bathing to health and fitness. Although they might not agree on whether a daily bath was necessary or what the water temperature should be, they convinced Americans that one could not be dirty and healthy at the same time.[23]

By the middle of the nineteenth century, health reformers and household manuals asserted that not only water but also soap was necessary for complete personal cleanliness. In the early nineteenth century soap manufacturers were producing a harsh product suitable for laundering and scouring and perfumers were producing luxury toilet soap for the complexions of wealthy women. Gradually, however, soap manufacturers began to mass produce toilet soap suitable for cleaning the skin and to advertise both their products and the importance of personal cleanliness. By 1885 the Reverend Henry Ward Beecher was advertising Pear's Soap, announcing that "if Cleanliness is next to Godliness Soap must be considered as a Means of Grace and a Clergyman who recommends moral things should be willing to recommend Soap."[24]

The fact that American middle- and upper-class standards of personal cleanliness were diverging from those of the poor and that cleanliness had taken on a symbolic meaning, also greatly increased demand for public baths. By mid-nineteenth century, as Claudia and Richard Bushman maintained, "Among the middle class anyway, personal cleanliness ranked as a mark of moral superiority and dirtiness as a sign of degradation. Cleanliness indicated control, spiritual refinement, breeding; the unclean were vulgar, coarse, animalistic."[25] In the face of squalid urban slums and the threat of epidemics, particularly cholera, these new standards of cleanliness led to the first formal investigations of the public health of cities and to recommendations for sanitary reform, including the provision of public baths.

The conditions of the slums in which immigrants lived were revealed by investigations undertaken mostly by physicians. John Griscom, a New York city inspector, in his eloquent and comprehensive report, *The Sanitary Condition of the Laboring Population of New York* (1845), revealed the horrors of slum life. Describing the housing available to the poor, Dr. Griscom wrote, "Every corner of the room . . . is piled up with dirt. The walls and ceilings, with plaster broken off in many places, . . . leaving openings for the escape from within of the effluvia of vermin dead and alive, are smeared with the blood of unmentionable insects and dirt of all indescribable colors . . . the chimneys [are] filled with soot, the whole premises populated thickly with vermin, the stair-ways . . . [are] the receptacle for all things noxious." He cited the very high mortality rates among the foreign born and their children, for which he blamed the vile and unhealthy environment that surrounded them. In Boston, Lemuel Shattuck, an amateur statistician, reported similarly shocking mortality figures from 1845 on.[26]

The 1849 cholera epidemic which ravaged American cities also produced increasing demands for cleanliness and for public baths. In this year Milwaukee built special bathhouses for newly arrived immigrants. Even more significantly, in this same year the Committee on Public Hygiene of the newly organized American Medical Association urged the establishment of cheap public baths on the European model in the parts of the cities inhabited by the lower classes. Specifically surveying the cities of Philadelphia and Baltimore, the committee found that although Philadelphia had five commercially operated public baths, these were too expensive for the poor. The only baths available to the poor were furnished by "one benevolent institution" established to supply employment to the poor. They provided hot and cold baths for three cents each or the equivalent in labor. The committee found no public baths in Baltimore, although it noted that in that city "an appendage to a fashionable house is invariably a bath-room."[27]

Although the American Medical Association committee felt (rather prophetically, considering the fate of American public baths) that "public baths are no proper substitute for the private bath-room in one's own dwelling," it apparently concluded that this was not possible for the poorer classes and that public baths were the answer. In arguing for public baths, the committee asserted that frequent bathing among the poor and laboring classes would remove "a prominent cause of disease and contribute to [their] moral, as well as physical improvement." It also stated: "That uncleanliness and mental degradation are intimately associated with each other, is now generally admitted; hence, in proportion as the body is kept cleanly, are the moral faculties elevated, and the tendency to commit crime diminished." These arguments foreshadow those later put forward by the bath advocates of the Gilded Age and the Progressive Era. In the 1840s and later, urban reformers saw the slum not only as a threat to social stability but also as a symptom of the moral depravity of slum dwellers. Cleanliness would produce higher moral standards in the slums.[28]

Another recommendation that cities establish public baths for the poor came from the Massachusetts Sanitary Commission of 1850. This commission reported that there were twelve or more commercial bathhouses in Boston charging from 12½ to 25 cents per bath, a price far too costly for the lower classes.[29]

A somewhat different point of view was presented in an 1846 article in *DeBow's Review* written by a New Orleans physician. Advocating a revival of municipal baths in the ancient Roman style, the author stressed the importance of regular bathing to health and deplored the lack of public baths: "Modern nations have borrowed from the ancient Romans almost everything worth borrowing except their magnificent baths. Such a thing as a public bath, erected at the public expense, and free to all without charge or for only a mere pittance is quite unknown in these modern times." He urged that New Orleans and other cities build public baths like the Roman thermae which would not only promote the health of their citizens but would be "a splendid ornament to the city" as well.[30]

No city governments responded to these demands for public baths. Pre–Civil War cities were just beginning to expand and regularize their municipal services as they established water and sewage systems, police and fire departments. Many services were left to private enterprise, such as urban transit and street cleaning. And it was a private charitable organization, the New York Association for Improving the Condition of the Poor (AICP), that built the first public bath for the poor. This city-wide organization had been founded in 1843 in response to conditions magnified by the Panic of 1837 and was the prototype for similar organizations founded in other major cities. Although the AICP reformers tended to blame slum conditions on the degraded moral character of the poor, they also recognized that the physical conditions of the slums could deepen moral failures and contaminate innocent children. Therefore, in addition to attempting to transmit moral values to the poor, the AICP worked for a panoply of public health and environmental reforms usually associated with the Progressive Era, such as medical dispensaries, better housing, pure milk, and public baths.[31]

In 1849 the AICP was authorized by the state legislature to incorporate the People's Bathing and Washing Association for the purpose of building a public bath. As a result of AICP efforts, the People's Bathing and Washing Establishment was opened at 141 Mott Street on the Lower East Side in 1852. This bathhouse cost $42,000 and included laundry facilities, a swimming pool, and tub baths for males and females. The charge for the laundry was three cents per hour and baths cost from five to ten cents. The bath was open only in the summer months. "The object [was] to promote cleanliness and comfort among the poor, at the smallest possible cost—the prices barely paying the actual expense." This bath was greatly needed, for as Robert Ernst has observed: "When water for bathing and washing had to be fetched from street pumps or near-by wells, bodily cleanliness was more of an ideal than a reality. Not only was it impossible to bathe, but insufficient space and air hindered home laundering."[32]

The AICP at first deemed the bath a success, maintaining that "it greatly contributed to the health, cleanliness, and comfort of those for whom it was designed" and citing its patronage of nearly 60,000 persons yearly as satisfactory. In 1861, however, the AICP closed the People's Bathing and Washing Establishment and stated later that "the enterprise was too far in advance of the habits of the people . . . to be appreciated by them and hence it failed through insufficient patronage" and was not self-supporting. What they did not say was that the bath was probably too expensive for the poor it was supposed to serve. A few years after the establishment of the People's Bath a *Verein* (association) was formed to crusade for free baths for the German working population in New York City, but this venture also failed.[33]

The Civil War interrupted the movement for public baths but also had a significant effect on public health reform. The well-publicized work of the United States Sanitary Commission and its investigations of sanitary conditions in army hospitals reinforced the idea of the importance of cleanliness to health and the connection between filth and disease.[34]

After the Civil War, Americans concerned with urban slums were faced with constantly accelerating urban growth and new waves of immigration which made the slums more threatening. By 1900, for example, New York City's population was 3,437,202, of whom 37 percent were foreign born. Other cities in both the East and Midwest experienced similar spurts of growth. Labor unrest and frequent economic depressions added to the disorder and violence characteristic of post–Civil War cities, and city bosses assumed control of municipal governments. Yet, as Morton Keller has pointed out, Gilded Age urban social reformers were limited in their capacity to take remedial action against the slums. Their desire for governmental economy, their hostility to governmental activism, and their belief that the poor were responsible for their own condition or that poverty arose out of unalterable social or hereditary laws combined to inhibit effective action. The major exception to this limitation was the area of public health and a wave of sanitary reform swept Gilded Age cities.[35]

Although the provision of public baths was one of the goals of sanitary reformers, the public bath movement gained momentum slowly. Probably the key development prior to 1890 was the establishment by several municipalities of free open-air or enclosed summer bathing facilities along river- or oceanfronts. The erection and maintenance of these baths at public expense probably encouraged the bath proponents by paving the way for popular acceptance of the idea of more expensive year-round baths as a logical extension of municipal services.

In 1866 in Boston a joint committee of the common council and board of aldermen was appointed "to examine and report upon the practicability of establishing within this city one or more Bathing Places for the free accommodation of the public." At first it hoped to set up saltwater baths for the summer and warm and cold freshwater baths for the rest of the year. But the committee found that year-round baths would be too expensive and instead concentrated on summer baths. The sum of $10,000

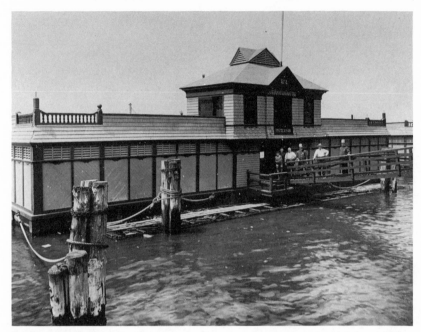

Exterior View, Floating Bath No. 2, New York City. Source: Community Service Society Papers, Rare Book and Manuscript Library, Columbia University.

was appropriated at first with another $10,000 added later. The committee then selected six locations for saltwater baths.[36]

In June 1866 Boston opened five floating baths at river sites and one natural beach bath (the L Street Bathing Beach). The floating baths were wooden, dock-like structures, the shape and depth of modern swimming pools, with dressing rooms located around the sides. Some of them had shallow areas for small children; river water was used to fill them. In their first summer of operation these baths were highly successful, recording a total of 433,690 bathers. Boston's total population at the time was approximately 200,000. In the next thirty years more of these baths were opened, and in 1897 Boston could boast 14 floating and beach baths operating under the supervision of the board of health. In placing these baths under this jurisdiction the municipal government was emphasizing that their purpose was to promote cleanliness, although the patrons probably considered them mainly recreational.[37]

New York City closely followed Boston's pioneering efforts in the provision of summer bath facilities. In its annual report for 1866 the

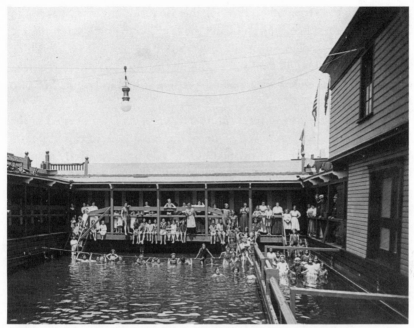

Girls' and Women's Day at a floating bath, New York City. Source: Community Service Society Papers, Rare Book and Manuscript Library, Columbia University.

board of health had urged the establishment of a system of free public baths, at the same time hoping that this would not "incur an unwarrantable expense to the municipal government." In the decade from 1868 to 1878 the New York State legislature passed a series of laws authorizing New York City to build floating baths to be located in the East and Hudson rivers and at the Battery. The first two floating baths were built and opened in 1870, and by 1888 the city had built and was operating under the Department of Public Works 15 floating baths. These baths cost an average of $9,500 each to build, and after 1888 an average of 2,500,000 males and 1,500,000 females used the baths yearly during the bathing season (approximately June 10 to October 1).[38]

New York's floating baths were free, were very popular among the poorer citizens of New York, and provided welcome relief from summer heat. There was a conflict, however, for the floating bath patrons considered them mainly a means of recreation, whereas the city authorities considered them a means to cleanliness and imposed a twenty-minute time limit for bathing. On hot summer days young boys often went from one floating bath to another, dirtying themselves on the way so as not to be denied admittance. Almost before the last floating bath was built, the problem of the pollution of the river water by sewage was reaching serious proportions. As a result, in 1914 all floating baths were required to be watertight, and if river water was used, it had to be purified and filtered.[39]

In Philadelphia also, several summer river baths were opened in the Gilded Age. In 1885, however, some of these baths were closed due to river pollution, and the city opened its first swimming pool. By 1899 the city of Philadelphia was operating eight such pools approximately 40 by 60 feet in size, but all its river baths had been closed because of pollution.[40]

The floating baths, beaches, and swimming pools, which were open only in the summer, did not solve the problem of the uncleanliness of the poor. They did, nevertheless, become an accepted part of the services a city should provide for its inhabitants. The next step, probably hastened by the pollution of the floating baths, was the provision of year-round bath facilities, which, as has been seen, had already been urged by the American Medical Association in 1849, the Massachusetts Sanitary Board in 1850, and the New York City Board of Health in 1866. In 1879 the *New York Daily Tribune* ran an editorial which urged "this great city" to establish year-round hot water baths, maintaining that, "every work of this nature is a direct benefit to the city. . . . A large proportion of the diseases which crowd our hospitals are engendered by uncleanliness much of which might be removed by effective public bathing facilities." In 1883 another *Tribune* editorial pressed for the construction of public baths, admitting that a municipal bath system would be costly but maintaining that the death rate would decrease and intemperance and immorality would be diminished. It suggested that a wealthy citizen might donate a bath to the city instead of a library, college, or art gallery. Such a person "could not choose a better or easier way by which not alone to keep their memories green, but to ameliorate the lot of their less fortunate fellows and to elevate and civilize both their contemporaries and posterity."[41]

While both these editorials met with no response from city officials or philanthropists in New York, a more official statement came from the Tenement House Committee of 1884, which had been created by the state legislature to investigate slum conditions in New York City. Among its recommendations was the following: "That the city shall establish free winter baths throughout the tenement house districts of the city. . . . Free winter baths would greatly enhance the cleanliness of the tenement house population, would lessen the danger of disease, and would be one safe-guard against the spread of epidemics."[42]

Although this recommendation too had no immediate effect, the way was paved for the bath reformers who would become more numerous and insistent in the 1890s. In this decade and the next the movement for public baths gained great momentum and the bath reformers saw their desires become reality, not only in New York but in many cities through-out the United States.

# 2

## Public Baths in the Progressive Era

Soap and water have worked a visible cure already that goes more
than skin deep. They are moral agents of the first value in the slum.
—JACOB A. RIIS

During the Progressive Era the public bath movement achieved its greatest success, as urban reformers, now far more numerous and exploiting
new weapons, renewed their efforts to solve the problems of America's
cities. Structural reformers sought to end boss rule by changing the structure of city governments and introducing better control of finances, business efficiency, and management by experts. The social reform urban
progressives pursued social justice, which they believed was most threatened by the urban slum, as already appalling conditions were exacer-
bated by the Depression of 1893 and its aftermath. To them, as to their
predecessors, the slum was, as Arthur Mann has pointed out, the epit-
ome of the primary evils of the day: "unemployment, racial and religious
prejudice, spiritual and physical want, class oppression, filth, disease,
prostitution, drink and corrupt politics." Not only was the slum an economic and sanitary problem, but also its very existence threatened the
social stability of the city as a whole.[1]

The social reform progressives were not consistent in their approach
to the problems of the slums. As Paul Boyer and others have observed,
they either adopted coercive and repressive strategies as exemplified by
their attacks on prostitution and the drinking of alcoholic beverages or
turned to "positive environmentalism," which would improve the surroundings of the poor and in so doing elevate their character and morality. These strategies were not mutually exclusive and many reformers ad-

vocated both types of reform. In both cases the reformers wished to exert social control over the slum population. The familiar litany of demands of the "positive environmentalists" included parks, playgrounds, kindergartens, tenement house regulation, public school reform, effective garbage collection and street cleaning, and public baths. Provision of these services by municipal governments would help to "humanize the city environment" and "redistribute at least in part some of the amenities of middle-class life to the masses" as well as give them an opportunity for "a decent life: that is, to be well fed and housed, to be clean, and to be moral human beings."[2]

The reasons that public baths were almost always included in this list of reforms are complex and illustrate several aspects of progressive reform motivation and its rhetoric. Although many of the arguments in favor of public baths in the Progressive Era echo those of bath advocates in the mid-nineteenth century and the Gilded Age, they also demonstrate the progressives' more sympathetic attitudes toward the poor. They tended to place less emphasis on the defective character of the poor as the main cause of poverty and also considered the effects of social and economic conditions and the slum environment.[3]

Obviously, public baths would provide for the poor a means of attaining personal cleanliness which their crowded tenements lacked. The progressives not only linked dirt with a poverty that grew out of individual habits of laziness, weakness, degeneration, or thriftlessness but also connected dirt to deficiencies in the environment in which the poor lived. The New York Tenement House Committee of 1894 (established by the state legislature to investigate slum conditions and successor to the 1884 committee of the same name) reported sympathetically that in New York City

the only way in which the occupants of tenement-houses can bathe is by using a tub of some kind, filled from the faucet in the kitchen or from that in the hall, or with water carried up from the yard. It is apparent that such conditions as these do not encourage the practice of bathing. Nor is this all. The number of rooms occupied by a family in a tenement-house is so small that every inch of space is occupied. Even when the occupants are willing to incur the labor of carrying water from the faucet in the hall or from the yard it is difficult to secure the privacy which is necessary for the bath.

The poor were perceived as dirty, bearers of the "tenement odor," not because of cultural variance from American middle-class bathing habits but because they lacked bath facilities. A New York City Health Department inspector wrote in 1884 that poverty and uncleanliness went hand in hand "because these poor people have not the facilities to keep themselves clean, . . . they have no baths."[4]

Growing acceptance of the germ theory of disease in the 1890s by both American physicians and the general public added a scientific argument and an increased urgency to the demand for public baths and brought more support to the movement from the medical profession. As medical researchers identified the bacteria responsible for diseases such as typhoid, tuberculosis, cholera, and diphtheria, sanitarians transferred their attention from the environment to the individual as a source of contagion and emphasized the importance of personal cleanliness.[5]

Noting that "the better situated classes" came in contact with the poor as employees, servants, laborers, tradespeople, and mechanics, Simon Baruch, a physician and foremost leader of the public bath movement, stressed that everyone's health would be protected if the poor were clean. More alarmingly, another physician and member of the board of health, Moreau Morris, warned his fellow New Yorkers that "the body exhalations of an unwashed sample of humanity sitting next to us in our crowded cars may communicate a deadly typhus germ without our consciousness." Although sanitary reformers did not abandon the effort to achieve a cleaner slum environment through effective garbage collection, street cleaning, sewer systems, and other means, they stressed the role played by the infected individual as a bearer of disease. For example, in urging the provision of public baths, the New York Tenement House Committee of 1894 reiterated: "Cleanliness is the watchword of sanitary science and the keynote of the modern advice aseptic surgery. If it apply to the street, the yard, the cellar, the house and the environment of men it most certainly should apply to the individual." By 1916, Charles Zueblin would write in *American Municipal Progress* that public baths were "an indispensable protection of the public health."[6]

Public bath advocates were not content with asserting that the provision of baths would guarantee the attainment of middle-class standards of bodily cleanliness among the poor and safeguard the public health; echoing their predecessors throughout the nineteenth century, they also stressed the salutary effects that cleanliness would have on the moral character of the poor. Writing in a United States government publication, G. W. W. Hanger stated that public baths would "stimulate in a powerful way a feeling of self-respect and a desire for self-improvement" and "elevate the material and moral tone of the poorer classes." Boston's mayor, Josiah Quincy, stated that "when physical dirt has been banished, a long step has been taken in the elimination of moral dirt." Bath reformers equated physical cleanliness with moral purity. As John Paton, president of the New York Association for Improving the Condition of the Poor, proclaimed, "With very large classes of society cleanliness of person, apparel and home are inseparable from thrift, industry and prosperity, and it is the absence of this which distinguishes upright, honest poverty from the condition of the improvident, the depraved and the worthless."[7] Public baths therefore would at the same time reform both the slum environment and the character of the individual.

Cleanliness was also extolled as one of the hallmarks of civilization and progress. Simon Baruch observed, "The civilizing influence of soap and water has long been recognized," and, recalling the opulent Roman baths as earlier bath reformers had, he declared, "It is a sad commentary on our boasted civilization" that we do not "emulate their generosity in supplying the poor with means for keeping their bodies clean and undefiled." Public baths would, he thought, assist in creating "civic civilization" out of "urban barbarism."[8]

Nativism, in a paternalistic but not xenophobic sense, also played a role in the rationale for public baths. The bath reformers asserted that the encouragement of regular bathing habits would assist in the Americanization and assimilation of the immigrant, and indeed most public baths were located in immigrant neighborhoods. They argued that one characteristic of immigrants which most emphasized their difference from the native-born was their lack of cleanliness. The *Brooklyn Daily Eagle* noted in a 1902 editorial calling for the building of municipal baths: "It is safe to say that some of our new citizens have never bathed since they came to America, and that others look upon a bath as a ceremonial to be indulged with caution . . . hence to be observed not oftener than once a year." Immigrants, the *Eagle* had asserted in an earlier editorial, must "be weaned from" their practice of not bathing "and made to comport themselves like self-respecting Americans." One bath reformer stated that the existence of public baths among the foreign element of all nationalities made them more cleanly in homes, shops, factories, and attire. Their children were less neglected and one no longer saw "dirty faces, unkempt hair and tattered and soiled clothing." A Chicago bath advocate was of the opinion that "the greatest civilizing power that can be brought to bear on these uncivilized Europeans crowding into our cities lies in the public bath."[9]

In spite of this nativist stereotype, not all immigrants were unwashed. Traditional religious ritual and social customs required that the Eastern European Jewish population bathe regularly. Although few Jewish families had bathing facilities in their dwellings, the number of privately owned bathhouses to serve them increased. Moses Rischin observed that in New York City, for example, "By 1897 over half of the city's sixty-two bath-houses (including Russian [steam], Turkish [hot air], swimming, vapor, and medicated bathhouses) were Jewish." The comparatively good health and low death rate among Jewish immigrants can probably be attributed in part to their standards of personal and home cleanliness. Although it might be expected that Jewish immigrants would be in the forefront of groups demanding the provision of public baths, they do not seem to have been particularly active, nor were other immigrant groups. Simon Baruch, although a Jew, was more interested in baths for reasons of public health than because of his Jewish background.[10]

Although the bath reformers claimed that public baths would change the moral character of the slum dweller and Americanize the immigrant, they never clearly explained how this would happen, nor did they seek to ascertain if the introduction of public baths actually produced any of the desired changes in the poor. They simply assumed that the poor and immigrants would change their ways once they were exposed to proper behavior in regard to bathing, and that other aspects of the American middle-class way of life would soon follow.

Bath reformers insisted that the solution to the problem of unclean-liness among the poor was a civic responsibility. The notion that slum landlords should be required to provide bathrooms for their tenants was generally disregarded. For example, although the Tenement House Law of 1901 in New York City did require private toilets, it did not require private bath facilities. In writing about this law, housing reformer Law-rence Veiller asserted that it was "felt that to require a private bath for each family as a matter of law, was not practicable and might with diffi-culty be sustained if attacked in the courts." It is probable that bath-rooms were considered too expensive to be included in low-rent private dwellings, and such a requirement might violate the property rights of owners. Bath reformers made only token efforts to urge private enterprise to provide bath facilities for the poor. A good example is a *New York Times* editorial which asked why the owners of tenement houses should not be compelled to provide these facilities but concluded that, if this could not or should not be done, it was the city's responsibility and not that of private charitable associations to provide this service for the needy. At the same time, the editorial counseled that "the city should confine itself to the erection of modest baths" which should be as close to "self-supporting" as possible.[11]

The ambivalent attitude of bath reformers toward the provision of private bath facilities can be further documented. In Baltimore, partly as a result of the bath movement, a law was passed requiring a bath to be built in every new house. This law, instead of being seen as a victory for bath advocates, invoked the following response from one New York bath leader: "Of what good is such a law unless it is followed by a clause compelling every man to take a bath at stated times? I say let us have public baths and still more public baths." The *Philadelphia North American* hoped for a future when "public baths will be as common as public schools, and bathing, like education, will be made compulsory." Obviously some bath reformers felt that the poor could not be trusted to bathe in the privacy of their own homes. This may be one reason that they never mentioned the alternative of paying higher wages to the poor, thus allowing them to afford homes equipped with baths. However, advocating higher wages, like requiring tenement house owners to provide bath facilities, would infringe on the property rights of landlords and employers, something the bath reformers were unwilling to do.[12]

The question of whether cities should spend the taxpayer's money to build public baths, which raised the issue of municipal socialism, appears not to have been seriously considered by the proponents of this reform, although an occasional dissenting voice was heard. In the opinion of the *Rochester Herald,* free baths would teach the people that they had a right to what they had not earned. "Gloss the matter as you may," the editor wrote, "the person who accepts a free public bath has accepted what another person has been compelled to pay for. In ethics it is no more honest than would be the theft of 25 cents spent on a bath in a private establishment." However, most contemporaries agreed with the *New York Daily Tribune* that this was a responsibility the city must accept. The failure of the city to build public baths, something that could be done by nobody else, was "little short of criminal," the editor asserted.

"The provision of baths and other conveniences is a proper municipal function, which should no more be neglected than street lighting or sewers." The Baltimore Bath Commission stated that public baths were no longer "a luxury nor charity, but a public necessity and obligation." Public baths, like parks and playgrounds, were becoming an essential part of the expanded number of services to be provided by municipal governments in this period.[13]

Further impetus to the bath movement came from the example of European cities as well as from civic pride and rivalry among American cities. Cultural deference in the form of imitation of European responses to urban problems often spurred and legitimatized urban reform in this era and the bath movement was no exception. As we have seen, many of the major European cities had municipal bath systems, and the American proponents of municipal baths frequently alluded to this. For example, the authors of the New York Tenement House Committee *Report* of 1894 wrote: "It would conduce greatly to the public health if New York should follow the example of many of the cities of the Old World and open municipal baths in the crowded districts." In 1897 the Mayor's Committee on Public Baths and Comfort Stations in New York reported that "New York and other American cities are far behind those of Europe, especially London, Birmingham, Glasgow, Paris and Berlin." Rivalry among American cities was reflected when advocates of public baths in Baltimore concluded that the Maryland city was lagging behind New York and Boston and urged it "to make a beginning without delay and to lay the foundations for a more elaborate [bath] system in the future."[14]

Not only was civic pride a factor in supporting the construction of municipal baths but it was also gratified once the bath system was a functioning reality. The Public Baths Association of Philadelphia boasted that its first bathhouse had been visited by representatives "from St. Louis, Chicago, New York, Baltimore and other leading cities, with the result of stimulating the bath-house movement throughout the country." The *Baltimore Sun* asserted that the city's portable baths "are making quite a sensation in the bath world, and other cities are talking of adopting them." The Baltimore Bath Commission stated that the successful management of its bath system has "given our city a national reputation in this department."[15]

Although no doubt existed in the minds of municipal bath advocates that there was great need for public bath facilities in the congested slum

Table 2.1.    Percent of Families and Individuals in Houses or
Tenements with Bathrooms, 1893[a]

| City | Percent of Families | Percent of Individuals |
|------|---------------------|------------------------|
| Baltimore | 7.35 | 9.21 |
| Chicago | 2.83 | 3.76 |
| New York | 2.33 | 6.51 |
| Philadelphia | 16.90 | 18.05 |

[a]Carroll D. Wright, *The Slums of Baltimore, Chicago, New York and Philadelphia,* 94.

areas of American cities, they, like most reformers of the Progressive Era, began to gather more facts and statistics to prove their claims. In 1887 Dr. George H. Rohé of Baltimore reported to the American Medical Association convention in Chicago that a large proportion of the inhabitants of American cities had no proper bathing facilities. In the 18 cities that he surveyed he found that only 23 percent of the residences were supplied with bathtubs. In Baltimore, of 70,000 houses, only 20,000 had bathtubs.[16]

In 1892 the chief of the Bureau of Statistics of the Labor Department of Massachusetts conducted a tenement house census in Boston. Studying 71,665 families renting tenements or apartments, he found that only 18,476 families (25.78 percent ) had bathrooms. In one of the slum wards (ward 6), fewer than 1 percent of the families had bathrooms, but in ward 11, exclusive Back Bay, 72.15 percent had bathrooms.[17]

Further proof of the lack of bath facilities came in 1893, when the Bureau of Labor, a federal agency, investigated the most congested slum districts in four major cities. Table 2.1 summarizes the results. By calling attention to the lack of bathing facilities in urban slums in this report, which was prepared in compliance with an 1892 congressional resolution, the federal government further legitimatized the bath movement and its concern with the lack of cleanliness of the poor. Subsequently it gave more support to the movement in 1901, when the Bureau of Labor and Commerce presented an exhibition on public baths in Europe at the Pan-American Exposition, and in 1903, when the same agency mounted an exhibition on public baths in the United States at the Louisiana Purchase Exposition. The federal government published extensive reports on each of these exhibits illustrated with photographs and floor plans of public baths. These exhibitions and reports not only publicized the bath movement but also gave it the official imprimatur of the federal government by emphasizing that baths were an essential part of city services.[18]

Statistics on the lack of bathing facilities continued to appear. In addition to recommending the building of public baths, the New York Tenement House Committee of 1894 reported that out of a population of 255,033 people, only 306 had access to bathrooms in their dwelling places. Another study of workingmen's families in New York, conducted in 1907, found that the number of families having bathrooms was directly proportional to family income (for example, in families with an annual income of $400–599, 4 percent had bathrooms and in those with incomes of $900–1,099, 24 percent had bathrooms). Of the entire group studied, however, only one family in seven had bathrooms.[19]

In *The Battle with the Slum* Jacob Riis gave more dramatic evidence of the lack of bath facilities in New York's slums. His photograph of a bathtub hanging under a tenement apartment window high above street level in an air shaft was captioned "The only Bath-tub in the Block" This block, a model of which was displayed at the Tenement House Exhibition of 1900 organized by the Charity Organization Society, contained two acres bounded by Chrystie, Forsyth, Canal, and Bayard streets. In its 39 tenements housing 2,781 persons, including 466 children under five, there were only 247 water closets and this one bathtub.[20]

The lack of bath facilities for urban slum dwellers cannot be disputed. What is in doubt is whether there was a "long-felt want" for public baths among the slum population. Even the public bath adherents themselves had to admit that where private bathtubs did exist in tenements, they often were not put to their proper use. As tenement landlords like to point out and tenement house inspectors had to agree, they often were used instead as storage areas, coal bins, and the like. This misuse of bathtubs may be attributed to the lack of hot water in tenements and the fact that the poor had not acquired the habit of bathing regularly. Public bath advocates, however, never asked whether slum dwellers wanted public baths. The assumption was that they did, and the fact that they failed to use private bathtubs when they had them only reinforced the idea that public baths were necessary.[21]

Seizing upon the example of European municipal baths, the statistical and other evidence of the need for public bathing facilities in American

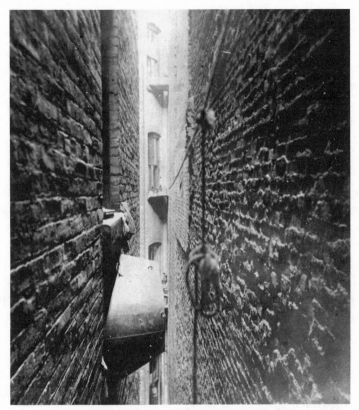

"The Only Bath-tub in the Block." Bathtub hanging below a tenement window in an air shaft, New York City. Source: Photograph by Jacob A. Riis, Jacob A. Riis Collection, Museum of the City of New York.

cities, and the impetus of the general reform attitude of Progressivism, American public bath advocates gathered their forces in the 1890s and met with little opposition and much support. Open disapproval of the municipal bath movement was rare, and the movement's worst enemy was indifference or apathy on the part of municipal governments and the general public.

Private philanthropy was often first in responding to the urgings of the bath advocates. In city after city public baths for slum dwellers were established first by private charitable organizations. The hope was that these baths would serve as a model and further illustrate the need for a municipal bath system. Settlement houses, for example, often provided limited bathing facilities for the neighborhoods they served. This was true of Hull House, the University of Chicago Settlement House, and of the University and College settlement houses in New York City. Settlement houses also took an active role in urging cities to supply municipal baths for slum dwellers, although baths were generally not high on their list of reform priorities.[22]

The largest and most influential prototype of the public bath was the People's Baths erected in New York City by the Association for Improving the Condition of the Poor in August 1891 at the urging of Simon Baruch. With John Wesley's maxim "Cleanliness Next to Godliness" inscribed above its door, this two-story building cost $27,025, raised through private contributions. It was located on the Lower East Side on land owned by the City Mission and Tract Society. It had 23 showers and three bathtubs; each bathing compartment was divided into a dressing room of 3½ by 4 feet and a shower area of the same size. Future baths followed this model. The five-cent fee, which included towel and soap, nearly covered operating expenses. The Colgate Company donated eighty pounds of soap to be distributed to patrons of the bath as free samples. The People's Baths were well patronized, furnishing 10,504 baths in 1891, 88,735 in 1895, and 115,685 in 1898. The baths received coverage in the New York and Boston press and were also publicized by the AICP itself. A local poet and physician, Gouverneur M. Smith, celebrated the opening of the bath and expressed the mixed motives and hopes of the bath reformers with these concluding verses:

> The man who is clean from his scalp to his toes,
> Should always be jolly, wherever he goes.
> To be clean without leads to pureness within.
> Where lurks germs, the vilest of terrible sin.
>
> So hurra! Yes, hurra! that this bathhouse is built.
> At sin and at filth to make a brave tilt.
> May the AICP by this right royal gift,
> Save many a soul now wrecked and adrift.

Dozens of bath advocates visited the People's Baths, as did official delegations from cities also planning to build municipal baths, such as Yonkers, New York; Trenton, New Jersey; and Boston. The privately sponsored Public Baths Association of Philadelphia also carefully inspected these baths. In New York City other private charitable associations quickly

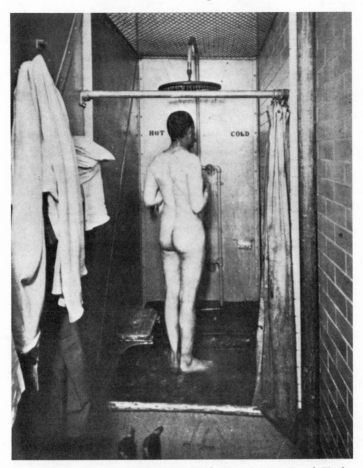

Bath Cubicle, People's Baths, New York City. Source: Frank Tucker, "Public Baths," in Robert W. DeForest and Lawrence Veiller, eds., *The Tenement House Problem*, vol. 2 (New York: Macmillan, 1903), between pp. 46 and 47. Economics and Public Affairs Division, New York Public Library, Astor, Lenox, and Tilden foundations.

followed the example of the AICP, and small public baths were opened under the auspices of the DeMilt Dispensary (1891), the Baron de Hirsch Fund (1892), the Cathedral Misson (1892), and the Riverside Association (1894).[23]

At the same time, some businesses began to supply bath facilities for their employees. In 1893, J. H. Williams and Company, an ironworks located in Brooklyn, modeled its bath, consisting of 12 showers, after the People's Baths and also provided laundry facilities where the workers could wash and dry their work clothes. Williams commented:

As it is acknowledged that habitual bathing prevents disease and promotes health and morality, baths for working people affect all classes of society. Employers are, therefore, under moral obligations to supply such facilities and health, decency and humanity demand it, because few opportunities for personal cleanliness are afforded to any but the privileged classes.

The Fifth Avenue Bank of New York provided bath facilities for its employees, as did the United Shoe Machinery Company of Boston. However, Parke, Davis and Company demurred, asserting that it had "found that good wages and short hours are preferred by the people to elaborately furnished toilet rooms, baths, gymnasia and similar devices."[24]

While gaining support and seeing their ideals becoming reality through private charity and business, public bath advocates could not agree among themselves as to what type of baths municipalities should build and whether the baths should be free or available at a minimal charge. Bath supporters did agree that shower baths were more efficient and easier to keep clean than tub baths, and almost all American public baths had showers rather than tubs. In this case Americans were following the German rather than the English example, for English baths usually contained more bathtubs than showers.[25]

The question that confounded bath reformers was whether public baths should be large, imposing, expensive, even monumental structures or small, simple, and unpretentious. European cities, especially in Germany, had built both types: small, inexpensive neighborhood people's baths that consisted mostly of showers, and large, monumental, centrally located municipal bathhouses that offered a variety of baths including showers, swimming pools, and even Turkish baths. Most American municipal bath advocates favored having many small, inexpensive public baths easily accessible to slum dwellers rather than the elaborate, expensive, centrally located bathhouse. This position was reiterated constantly, as in the federal government report written in 1901 by the Boston bath proponent Edward M. Hartwell:

Baths for the people should be centrally located in populous districts, where they are easily accessible. Numerous relatively small and comparatively inexpensive self-contained bath houses are vastly more desirable and useful than are struc-

tures of the costly monumental type for which architects and municipal coun-
cilors have too often shown so marked a predilection.[26]

Yet some cities succumbed to the temptation to erect bathhouses that
were also imposing public buildings. Boston's reform mayor Josiah Quincy defended this practice in his remarks at the formal opening of Boston's first bathhouse, which cost about $90,000:

> The expenditure which the city had made in erecting its first permanent bath
> house of this substantial and ornamental character had been incurred with a
> broader end in view than that of merely providing facilities for the bathing of a
> certain number of persons. The number of shower-baths and tub-baths con-
> tained in this building could have been furnished at a much smaller expense,
> and the city might, perhaps, have leased a building for the purpose, instead of
> purchasing a valuable lot of land and erecting an expensive structure. The
> purpose . . . was to erect a building of such character and appointments that it
> would be worthy as an architectural monument of the city which owned it, and
> would raise the whole idea of public bathing to a high and dignified plane.

The building of monumental municipal bathhouses was no doubt in part
a manifestation of the City Beautiful movement which swept through
American cities between 1890 and 1910. Basically, proponents of the city
beautiful believed that a more attractive, aesthetically pleasing, and im-
pressive urban environment would produce social cohesiveness and civic
loyalty and pride on the part of urban citizens. As a Boston resident put it,

> A city which does nothing except to police and clean the streets means little. But
> when it adds schools, libraries, galleries, parks, baths, lights, heat, homes and
> transportation, it awakens interest in itself. The citizen cares for the city which
> shows some care for him. He looks upon it as his city, and not a thing apart from
> him; and he becomes a good citizen because it is his city.[27]

Bath advocates also could not agree as to what facilities beyond shower
baths should be included in municipal bathhouses. Some insisted that
showers were all that was necessary. Others urged that swimming pools,
gymnasiums, or public laundries be included. American cities varied in
their responses to these demands. Chicago built simple bathhouses with
shower baths and little else. Baltimore and Philadelphia included public
laundries in their public bathhouses, whereas New York and Boston usually included swimming pools and gymnasiums, especially in bathhouses
built after 1900.[28]

Reformers also disagreed about whether municipal baths should be free or should charge a small fee. Some bath advocates felt that a small fee was "highly desirable as promoting a feeling of self-respect among the patrons . . . and an appreciation of the privileges afforded." Others felt that municipal baths should be absolutely free so that no one would be denied this privilege. Generally the public baths operated by private charitable institutions charged a minimal fee, usually five cents. Municipally operated baths, however, were usually free, and a New York State law required that city-owned baths could exact no fee. Nevertheless, a five-cent fee was often charged for soap and towel.[29]

Bath reformers also urged that shower baths be located in public schools either exclusively for the use of schoolchildren or for the use of the children during school hours and for the general public after school hours. There was some objection to this. For example, the Boston Schoolhouse Committee felt that it was not the duty of the school authorities "to bathe the children in the public schools because they may not be clean, for if this be granted, we see no reason why we should not clothe them if they be improperly clothed, or feed them if not properly nourished at home." These misgivings were overridden, however, and school baths were established in some of Boston's public schools. School baths were also built in public schools in New York City and Baltimore.[30]

Despite all these disagreements, the experience of using a public bath was remarkably similar throughout all bath systems. The baths were meant to be utilitarian and simply to furnish an opportunity for personal cleanliness. Generally a bath cubicle was divided into two parts—a dressing area and a shower, separated by a curtain. Men and women were strictly separated and order was stressed. Patrons were given a numbered check on entering the waiting room and, as cubicles were vacated, numbers were called. Usually twenty minutes were allowed for undressing, bathing, and dressing. Generally both the water temperature and the duration of the shower were controlled by bath attendants. Water temperature ranged from 73° to 105°F; anything hotter was thought to be "ennervating." Bath patrons apparently would have preferred to stay for longer than the allotted time, for a minor scandal erupted in New York City when officials discovered that attendants were permitting users who paid them five cents to use the baths as long as they wished. The guilty attendants were promptly dismissed.[31]

Many bath advocates also urged their cities to build public toilets, or comfort stations as they called them. Their main argument was that lack of such facilities forced men who worked outside, like policemen, into saloons. In New York and Baltimore bath reformers were instrumental in the establishment of public toilets. In general, however, bath reformers concentrated most of their interest and efforts on securing public baths and were only secondarily concerned with public toilets.[32]

After 1890 the municipal bath movement met with varying degrees of success in many American cities (see table 2.2). The first year-round municipal bath in the United States was the West Side Natatorium, which opened in Milwaukee in 1890. In this same year *Cosmopolitan* magazine held a competition offering a $200 prize for the best design of a public bath for the poor in a city of 100,000 population or more. The winning plan from over twenty submitted was for a monumental type of bath. It included separate men's and women's sections, with showers, bathtubs, and a swimming pool in each section plus a Turkish bath and a public laundry. *Cosmopolitan* advocated the building of public baths and set up a committee of its own editors and writers and some prominent New York citizens to seek ways of fulfilling this purpose. It also urged private philanthropists to consider the donation of a public bath: "It would be an American imitation of the noblest work of a Roman emperor—a truly imperial gift not out of keeping with the highest ambitions for the welfare of one's fellow citizens." There is no evidence, however, that *Cosmopolitan*'s bath committee succeeded at all in obtaining the construction of any public baths, although the publicity which the competition engendered probably aided the bath movement.[33]

As the 1890s progressed, several more cities built public baths. Chicago opened its first year-round bath in 1894. In 1895 impetus was added to the bath movement when the New York State legislature passed a law requiring all first- and second-class cities to build municipal baths. Yonkers promptly complied with this law, opening its first bath in 1896; Buffalo followed in 1897, and after some delay public baths were opened in Rochester in 1899, in Syracuse in 1900, and in Albany, Troy, and New York City in 1901.[34]

Brookline, Massachusetts, an affluent Boston suburb, opened what was probably the only public bath for the middle class in 1897. The bath was large and elaborate and had a sizable swimming pool (26 by 80 feet) as well as showers and tubs. It was built by the city after agitation led by a local physician and cost about $60,000. The Brookline bath received quite a bit of publicity and was considered "one of the most perfect in the country."[35]

Table 2.2.  Year-round Public Baths in the United States, 1904[a]

| | Population 1900 | | Bathhouses | | Total Number of | | | | Total No. of Baths for Year[c] | Free or Fee | Total Cost of Land and Buildings | Yearly Cost: Maintenance and Operation[c] |
|---|---|---|---|---|---|---|---|---|---|---|---|---|
| | Total | Percent Foreign Born | Total No. | Year Opened | Showers | Tubs | Swimming Pools | Laundries | | | | |
| I. Municipally operated | | | | | | | | | | | | |
| Albany | 94,151 | 18.8 | 1 | 1901 | 8 | 2 | 1 | 0 | 44,044 | Both[g] | $38,390 | $6,060 |
| Baltimore | 508,957 | 13.5 | 2 | 1900 | 49 | 4 | 0 | 2 | 150,925 | 3¢ | 70,950 | 11,590 |
| Boston | 560,892 | 35.1 | 10 | 1897 | 204 | 11 | 1 | 0 | 603,184 | Free | 794,200 | 58,500 |
| Brookline, Massachusetts | 19,935 | 32.7 | 1 | 1897 | 15 | 3 | 1 | 0 | 54,735 | 5–25¢ | 61,000 | 8,198 |
| Buffalo | 352,387 | 29.6 | 2 | 1897 | 50 | 2[b] | 0 | 0 | 194,650 | Free | 33,765 | 6,863 |
| Chicago | 1,698,575 | 34.6 | 7 | 1894 | 139 | 4 | 0 | 1 | 552,922 | Free | 76,092 | 18,042 |
| Cleveland | 381,768 | 32.6 | 1 | 1904 | 37 | 2 | 0 | 1 | [d] | [d] | 28,100 | [d] |
| Louisville, Kentucky | 204,731 | 10.5 | 1 | 1902 | 12 | 2 | 0 | 0 | 14,139 | Free | 5,400 | 1,440 |
| Milwaukee | 285,315 | 31.2 | 3 | 1890 | 53 | 13 | 3 | 0 | 576,625 | Free | 113,882 | 11,000 |
| New York | 3,437,202 | 37.0 | 5 | 1901 | 405 | 38 | 0 | 0 | 776,917[e] | Free | 502,617 | 34,000[e] |
| Portland, Maine | 50,145 | 20.8 | 1 | 1901 | 11 | 0 | 0 | 0 | 30,000 | Free | 2,357 | 1,200 |
| Rochester, New York | 162,608 | 25.1 | 1 | 1899 | 15 | 0 | 0 | 0 | 53,000 | Free | 15,500 | 3,000 |
| Syracuse, New York | 108,374 | 21.9 | 1 | 1900 | 16 | 20 | 1 | 0 | 69,667 | Free | 12,000 | 3,343 |
| Troy, New York | 60,651 | 23.7 | 1 | 1901 | 24 | 2 | 0 | 1 | 74,092 | Free | 14,000 | 1,800 |
| Yonkers, New York | 47,931 | 30.5 | 2 | 1896 | 46 | 4 | 0 | 0 | 25,169 | 5¢ | 22,315 | [h] |
| II. Nonmunicipally operated | | | | | | | | | | | | |
| Allegheny, Pennsylvania | 129,896 | 23.3 | 1 | 1903 | 20 | 8 | 0 | 0 | 20,021 | 5¢ | 87,000 | 2,000 |
| New York | 3,437,202 | 37.0 | 2 | 1891 | 54 | 3 | 0 | 0 | 162,638 | 5¢ | 27,025[f] | 8,396 |
| Philadelphia | 1,293,697 | 22.8 | 3 | 1898 | 75 | 9 | 0 | 2 | 62,377[f] | 5¢ | 61,142 | 5,002[f] |
| Pittsburgh, Pennsylvania | 321,768 | 26.4 | 2 | 1897 | 42 | 6 | 1 | 0 | 109,792 | 5¢ | 55,000 | 4,009 |
| San Francisco | 342,782 | 34.1 | 2 | 1890 | 0 | 60 | 1 | 0 | 125,000[f] | 10–50¢ | 55,719[f] | 7,969 |

[a]Hanger, 1254–61; U.S. Census Office, *Twelfth Census of the United States: 1900, Population*, 1:lxix.
[b]For infants.
[c]Year of figures varies from 1902 to 1904 depending on fiscal years.
[d]Recently opened.
[e]No figures for four baths recently opened.
[f]One bath only; the others not reported.
[g]Free 3 days per week to residents; other days, residents 10 cents, non-residents 25 cents.
[h]Not reported.

Boston's first year-round bath was opened in 1898 and Baltimore's in 1900. Cities as diverse as Portland, Maine, and Louisville, Kentucky, opened modest municipal baths in 1901 and 1902, respectively. Even the city of Davenport, Iowa (population about 36,000), was urged in 1901 to build a public bath and swimming pool for its working-class population because it was "advancing beyond the country-town period and entering the progressive-city stage." By 1904, a total of 15 cities had at least one municipally operated year-round public bath; and 18 other cities were operating summer baths such as swimming pools, floating baths, or beaches.[36]

Private philanthropy also continued to be active in the public bath movement in the 1890s. In 1890 the James Lick Bath was opened in San Francisco, followed by New York City's People's Baths in 1891. In 1897 the People's Baths of Pittsburgh were opened. Donated by Mrs. William Thaw, Jr., as a memorial to her husband, they were operated by the Civic Club of Allegheny County. The Public Baths Association of Philadelphia produced that city's first year-round bath in 1898 after raising funds in a city-wide campaign. In Allegheny, Pennsylvania, Henry Phipps donated a bathhouse in 1903 which was operated by the Public Wash House and Bath Association.[37]

Of the ten largest cities in the United States in 1900, only two, Saint Louis and Cincinnati, did not have either municipally or charitably operated year-round baths by 1904. In the decade of 1900–10 the municipal bath movement reached its peak as cities which already had baths built more, and new cities were added to the number which had municipal baths (Saint Louis opened its first bath in 1907). By 1922, more than 40 cities operated municipal year-round baths. Of the cities with large bath systems, Baltimore reported that it had 11 public baths (including school baths), Boston 12, Chicago 20, and New York City 25. Western cities, such as Denver, Omaha, and Salt Lake City, and southern cities, such as Dallas, Mobile, and Nashville, also had one or two public baths.[38]

There was no generally accepted way of administering municipal bath systems. The bath reformers felt that an unpaid bath commission composed of public-spirited men and women appointed by the municipal government to administer the bath system was the best solution. The bath commission usually appointed a full-time paid secretary who was responsible for the day-to-day supervision of the system. The bath systems of Baltimore and Boston were administered by this type of commission. In other cities there was wide variation. Buffalo's bath system was under the jurisdiction of the Department of Health, while Yonkers' was under the Department of Public Works. Saint Louis' baths were operated by the Public Recreation Commission. New York City's baths were at first operated by the Department of Public Buildings, Lighting and Supplies and later were transferred to the Public Works Departments in offices of the borough presidents.[39]

To the bath reformers a standard of cleanliness was necessary for participation in the common urban community. The "great unwashed" were a menace to the public health and moral well-being of their cities. Public baths would remove this danger and would help to make cities decent, healthful, safe, and enjoyable places to live.[40]

In the following chapters we will turn to detailed case studies of the actual process of how and why the public bath movement achieved success in five American cities. This achievement reveals the interrelationships of social reformers and urban governments as the nation moved from the Gilded Age into the Progressive Era. Public bath leaders, municipal governments and their officials (both bosses and reformers), state legislators, private philanthropists, and some of the slum dwellers themselves all played roles in each of these cities as they acted out the complex process of urban reform.

# 3

## Tammany Hall versus Reformers: The Public Baths of New York City

Reform in the Progressive Era was not always the product of mass protest movements as many have described it in the past, but of a relatively small group of people who saw possibilities of "social engineering" through organized and bureaucratic effort, private as well as public.

—SAMUEL P. HAYS

### The Campaign for Municipal Baths in New York City, 1887–1900

The quotation at the head of this chapter very aptly applies to the events leading up to the building of public baths in New York City, for this reform was largely the result of actions taken by private individuals and a variety of charitable organizations whose agitation for more than a decade finally forced the city government to take action. The impetus came neither from the city government itself nor from the tenement dwellers for whose benefit the baths were built. Bath advocates were most successful with the New York State legislature, and the history of the public bath movement from 1887 to 1901 (when the first municipal bath was opened) is that of a struggle to force city authorities to implement existing legislation.

The antibath forces do not appear as an organized group. In fact, the only group which actively opposed the building of public baths was the owners of commercial bathing establishments, and they were few. Successive city administrations under control of the Tammany Hall Democratic machine in the 1890s were not interested in building public baths and were largely responsible for the delay in the implementation of legislation. Public baths were not a major vote-getting issue, and the lack of popular ground swell in favor of them probably accounts for Tammany's lack of interest. Only under the reform administration of Mayor William L. Strong (1895–97) did the construction of the first municipal baths begin, and even during this period there were delays and misunderstandings.

As we have seen, the construction of floating baths in New York City, beginning in 1868, paved the way for demands that the city build year-round baths. Sporadically during the 1880s, the press, the Tenement House Committee of 1884, and the New York State legislature all recommended the establishment of free year-round baths to no avail. However, by the beginning of the 1890s the leadership of the bath movement had emerged and solidified and the effort began to achieve some success.[1]

New York City Progressives in general (the settlement-house workers, those involved in charitable organizations, and the anti-Tammany coalition of business and professional groups) favored the municipal provision of public baths, but baths were not high on their list of reform priorities. Settlement houses and other charitable organizations, for example, often provided a few shower baths for the public, but all these organizations were more active in promoting reforms other than public baths. To these reformers the need to root out corruption in urban government and correct more life-threatening slum conditions took precedence over the provision of public baths.

The leaders of the bath movement were more single-minded and worked primarily for the achievement of this one reform. In New York, Simon Baruch was the foremost individual bath advocate; the charitable organization, the New York Association for Improving the Condition of the Poor, lent its early and continuous support. On the state level, Goodwin Brown furnished the necessary leadership. The New York City press and physician's organizations also consistently supported the cause. In most American cities women played an important role in the public bath movement, but this did not occur in New York.

Simon Baruch, usually acknowledged as "the father of the public bath movement in the United States" and also the father of the more famous Bernard, was born in Germany and emigrated to South Carolina while in his teens. A regular, or orthodox, physician, he was awarded an M.D. degree by the Medical College of Virginia in 1862. He immediately joined the Confederate army as an assistant surgeon and served actively until the end of the Civil War. He settled in Camden, South Carolina, and practiced medicine there until 1881, when he moved to New York City. Baruch became prominent in 1888, when he successfully operated in a case he had diagnosed as appendicitis. This was supposedly the first time this operation had been performed in America and became standard treatment thereafter. He was best known, however, as a leading exponent of hydrotherapy and was the author of two standard texts on the subject, *The Uses of Water in Modern Medicine* (1892) and *The Principles and Practice of Hydrotherapy* (1898). He was also professor of hydrotherapy at the College of Physicians and Surgeons of Columbia University. Baruch was not interested only in hydrotherapy but wrote in medical journals on a variety of topics including malarial fevers and strychnine poisoning. A bibliography of his works runs to thirty-two pages.[2]

The step from hydrotherapy to municipal bath advocacy was a logical one. Baruch became interested in the cause of public baths after a European trip in the late 1880s during which he was greatly impressed by the German municipal bath systems. From this point onward Baruch devoted more and more of his time to the cause of public baths. He was one of the founders of the American Association for Promoting Hygiene and Public Baths and served as its president from its inception in 1912 until his death in 1921. He wrote: "I consider that I have done more to save life and prevent the spread of disease in my work for public baths than in all my work as a physician."[3]

The background of Goodwin Brown, the state's other leading bath advocate, was quite different from that of Simon Baruch. Born in Henderson, New York, in 1852, Brown was a graduate of Cornell University and practiced law in Buffalo. As a member of the newly established State Lunacy Commission in 1889, Brown became interested in public baths. After introducing shower baths in state institutions for the insane, Brown was the leading force in ensuring passage of the New York State municipal bath laws of 1892 and 1895 by the state legislature. In a series of letters to New York City newspapers in 1900 Brown claimed sole credit for the passage of these laws, although he and Baruch had apparently conferred as early as 1892.[4]

Inspired by the European example, Baruch began his campaign for municipal baths in New York City in the late 1880s and early 1890s. He was responsible for the shower baths set up in the New York Juvenile Asylum and was active in addressing medical societies, the board of health, and other groups on the need for public baths. He succeeded first in interesting the New York Association for Improving the Condition of the Poor, which built the very successful People's Baths on the Lower East Side, which opened in August 1891.[5]

Baruch also approached the Tammany-controlled city government in 1891 but was rebuffed by Mayor Hugh Grant. He then communicated with Alderman Henry Flegenheimer, who already had indicated his interest in the cause of public baths by offering in the *New York Sun* to open a subscription for this purpose by donating $250. Although nothing had come of Flegenheimer's offer, he and Baruch were able to persuade the board of aldermen on May 11, 1891, to pass a resolution "appropriating $25,000 for an experimental Rain Bath, and asking the Mayor to appoint a committee of three to supervise its construction." However, after several interviews with Mayor Grant, Flegenheimer stated that the mayor would "not act in the matter unless pushed to it by an overwhelming public sentiment," so nothing came of this resolution.[6]

A year later, the efforts of New York City's bath advocates produced a response in the New York State legislature. Under the leadership of Goodwin Brown enabling legislation (Chapter 473), which authorized any city, village, or town to establish free public baths and to make expenditures for this purpose, was passed in May 1892. This law remained a dead letter and was never implemented by New York City.[7]

The election of Thomas F. Gilroy as mayor of New York City in 1892 gave the bath advocates some hope, even though he was associated with Tammany Hall. He had been commissioner of public works and was closely identified with the very popular floating baths, but as mayor he was no more responsive than Grant had been. Again the bath reformers turned to the state legislature. In February 1893 Assemblyman Otto Kempner, after consultation with Baruch and New York City's health commissioner, introduced in the legislature a bill to establish a bureau of public baths in the city of New York and to provide for the construction and maintenance of six permanent public baths.[8]

Once more the opposition of Tammany obstructed the realization of bath reform. In March 1893 Baruch urged Mayor Gilroy to support Kempner's bill, which had no hope of passage if it was opposed by the mayor. The *New York Times* and *Evening Telegram* endorsed the bill editorially and many physicians favored it. However, Baruch reported, "I cannot say that Mayor Gilroy was especially impressed. He said he believed there was no public sentiment in favor of such baths." At committee hearings on the bill, city authorities were "bitterly opposed" to it and the bill was not reported out of committee. The reasons for this opposition are obscure, but most likely public apathy and fiscal restraint played a role.[9]

The years 1894 and 1895, however, marked a turning point for New York City's public bath movement. The bath reformers had done little specifically to produce this change, although their earlier work had its influence. It was rather the result of a wave of revulsion against Tammany government, which prompted a general city reform movement beneficial to all reform—including the cause of public baths. The reforming spirit of 1894 began in February, when the Republican-controlled legislature formed a committee to investigate New York City's police department. The crusading Reverend Charles H. Parkhurst had already charged the department with blackmail, extortion, and corruption. These charges were largely substantiated by the Lexow Committee hearings, which also traced the close connection between the police department and Tammany Hall.[10]

In May 1894 the state legislature established another committee to inquire into conditions in New York City. This was the Tenement House Committee of 1894, whose chairman was Richard Watson Gilder, former editor of *Scribner's Monthly* and well-known reformer. The committee's careful and factual study of the appalling conditions in New York City's slums had a significant effect on the municipal bath movement. As has already been noted, the committee found that in a slum population of 255,033 people only 306 had access to bathrooms in their dwelling places and also found that the year-round public bath facilities available to this slum population were meagre. Stressing the importance of cleanliness to health and to the prevention of disease, the committee asserted that the fact that "several hundred thousand people in the city have no proper facilities for keeping their bodies clean is a disgrace to the city and to the civilization of the nineteenth century." The committee's *Report* to the state legislature recommended that, "in addition to the free floating baths, maintained in the summer months, the city should open in the crowded districts fully equipped bathing establishments, on the best European models, and with moderate charges."[11]

In September 1894, the anti-Tammany forces in New York City began to unite for the purpose of electing a reform mayor. Good government clubs, the German American Reform Union, the Chamber of Commerce of the State of New York, anti-Tammany Democrats, Protestant moral reformers, Protestant and Jewish charity trustees, and Republicans were included among the members of New York City's elite who put together the Committee of Seventy. Formed as a result of a Madison Square Garden mass meeting on September 6, 1894, of a "representative body of citizens," the committee's purpose was to take "advantage of the present state of public feeling to organize a citizens' movement for the government of the City of New York, entirely outside of party politics and solely in the interest of efficiency, economy, and the public health, comfort and safety." The chairman of the Committee of Seventy was Joseph Laroque, a former president of the city's bar association, prominent member of the chamber of commerce, and mugwump. Members included J. Pierpont Morgan, investment banker Jacob Schiff, Gustav Schwab of the North American Lloyd Steamship Company, Carl Schurz, Elihu Root, former reform mayor Abram S. Hewitt, and the Reverend Charles Parkhurst.[12]

The Committee of Seventy was organized into executive and financial committees, and a series of subcommittees were set up to attack specific city issues, such as street cleaning, garbage disposal, small parks, public schools, tenement house reform, and public baths and lavatories. In addition, the platform of the Committee of Seventy included a call for "the establishment of adequate Public Baths and Lavatories for the promotion of cleanliness and increased public comfort, at appropriate places throughout the city."[13]

The Committee of Seventy's first task was to select a mayoral candidate to run against Hugh J. Grant, the Tammany candidate. Its choice was one of its own members, William L. Strong, a millionaire businessman, banker, and former president of the Business Men's Republican Club. Strong won the mayoral election of 1894 in a substantial victory for New York City's coalition of reformers. The work of the Committee of Seventy, however, did not stop with this success. After the election, in early 1895, the subcommittees began to issue their reports.[14]

The members of the Sub-Committee on Baths and Lavatories were men of varied backgrounds. The chairman was William Gaston Hamilton, a grandson of Alexander Hamilton and a retired businessman who had been chairman of the People's Baths Committee of the Association for Improving the Condition of the Poor. The vice-chairman was Moreau Morris, a physician who had long been interested in public health, having served in the 1860s and 1870s as health commissioner and as superintendent of New York City's health department and was still serving as a sanitary inspector with the health department. Morris had also served as a member of the Tenement House Committee of 1884, which had unsuccessfully recommended the building of public baths. William H. Tolman, the secretary of the subcommittee, was a professional reformer, general agent for the AICP, and secretary of the Reverend Charles Parkhurst's City Vigilance League. Later in his career he organized, with Josiah Strong, the League for Social Service (later the American Institute of Social Service). He was also the author of several books, including *Municipal Reform Movements in the United States, The Better New York,* and *Social Engineering.*[15]

The three other members' interest in the issue of public baths is less clear. James P. Archibald was a prominent labor and political leader. Born in Ireland, he migrated to the United States at the age of twenty and had become a paperhanger. In 1894 he was president of the Brotherhood of Paper Hangers and Decorators and secretary of the Central Labor Union. Active in politics, he had been a member of the United Labor party, the People's Municipal League, and the Henry George movement, and was an anti-Tammany Democrat and president of the Democratic Association of Workingmen of Greater New York. As a representative of labor, Archibald was an important member of the Committee of Seventy. Another member was John P. Faure, secretary of the Committee of Seventy. A businessman, he was active in charitable work and was chairman of the Floating Hospital, St. John's Guild. In 1895 Mayor Strong appointed him commissioner of Charities and Correction. The other member was David H. King, Jr., a socially prominent contractor who built Madison Square Garden and the Washington Arch.[16]

It is not clear why Simon Baruch was not a member of the Sub-Committee on Public Baths and Lavatories. Logically he should have been a member and he was eager to serve. John P. Faure, secretary of the Committee of Seventy, called on him in November 1894, after Strong's victory, and apparently informally invited him to become a member. Yet in the end, Baruch's membership was officially rejected, probably because of his identification with the regular Democratic party.[17]

The Sub-Committee on Baths and Lavatories issued its fifteen-page *Preliminary Report* in early 1895. The report began by asserting that New York City was lagging far behind European and other American cities in the building of baths and urged that the city begin immediately to remedy the situation. It recommended that the city build modest bathhouses on 25 by 100-foot lots, each equipped with 40 shower baths and public laundry facilities, and suggested six sites in tenement neighborhoods. It felt that this would be preferable to "two or three great bathing institutions costing large sums of money." The subcommittee further recommended that the city equip public schools with baths and requested that the architects of the People's Baths, Cady, Berg, and See, submit a plan for a bathhouse.[18]

Bath advocates, in addition to support from the Strong administration, achieved another major victory on April 21, 1895, when the New York State legislature passed a law (Chapter 351) making the establishment of public baths mandatory for all first- and second-class cities in the state (at that time, New York City, Brooklyn, Buffalo, Rochester, Syracuse, Troy, and Utica). The local board of health was to determine the number of baths necessary, baths were to be kept open fourteen hours per day, and hot and cold water were to be provided. This law, which was framed by Goodwin Brown, passed without difficulty. The background of its passage is obscure, and seemingly it had no direct connection with the Committee of Seventy, except that perhaps the Republican-controlled legislature wanted to assist the newly elected Republican mayor of the City of New York in producing demanded reforms.[19]

In July 1895, Mayor Strong began to take action on the question of municipal baths. The Committee of Seventy had disbanded on June 19, but on July 5 the mayor requested that the Sub-Committee on Baths and Lavatories reconstitute itself as the Mayor's Committee to continue its investigations and make further recommendations. The membership of the Mayor's Committee, therefore, was identical to that of the subcommittee except for John P. Faure, who did not serve because he had been appointed commissioner of Charities and Correction. The creation of the Mayor's Committee received wide coverage in the New York press, which for the first time showed a sustained interest in the municipal bath movement, not only in its editorial pages but also in reports on the preliminary recommendations of the committee and feature articles on the already existing public baths operating under charitable auspices.[20]

The Mayor's Committee, although not issuing its final report until 1897, quickly made preliminary recommendations which were substantially the same as those of its original Committee of Seventy report. However, it did upgrade its recommendation on the type of bath to be built, suggesting a 50 by 100-foot lot and a building containing 80 baths rather than 40. The secretary of the committee, William H. Tolman, recommended that the majority of the bath facilities (about 75 percent) should be subject to a fee and the remainder be free. Although the mandatory bath law required that municipal baths be free, Tolman contended that "a bath is not a charity . . . but should be a municipal provision for cleanliness on the payment of a fair charge. Then the user retains his independence."[21]

With these recommendations, New York began to implement the mandatory bath law of 1895. In August of that year, the board of health approved plans for a large bathhouse and the city began to search for a site as well as for the necessary appropriation. What followed, however, was an almost comic series of delays which prevented the opening of New York City's first municipal bath until 1901.[22]

The first cause of delay was the passage by the state legislature in March 1896 of an additional bath law (Chapter 122) which empowered the city to issue $200,000 worth of consolidated stock to cover the cost of public baths and authorized the city to locate public baths and toilets "in any public park of the City of New York." Mayor Strong had apparently requested this last provision to save the city the expense of buying land for bathhouses and comfort stations.[23]

A site was selected on Tompkins Square Park on the Lower East Side, but this choice resulted in strong opposition from the residents of this predominantly German and Irish neighborhood, who held an indignant meeting on May 26, 1896, protesting the construction of a public bath on this site. The *New York Daily Tribune* reported that the residents, in "proceedings . . . of a vehement, impassioned and turbulent nature," asserted that there was no need for a bath to be located there and suggested a site farther to the south on the Lower East Side, where the residents were newer Jewish and Italian immigrants. Tompkins Square residents felt further that locating a public bath in their park (which was small and the only park in the area) would "ruin the enjoyment" of those using the park for recreation and would be a detriment rather than a gain for their neighborhood. Although they did not actually state it, these people were rejecting the idea that they were so poor that they needed a public bath. They then appointed a committee, which included their alderman, assemblyman, and the pastor of the local Roman Catholic church, to testify at a meeting of the board of aldermen to be held the next day, where the Mayor's Committee on Public Baths and Lavatories was to make a report. Although the representatives of the neighborhood did not have the opportunity to speak, their opposition had its effect; they were joined by the editorial voice of the *New York Times*, which affirmed that the city needed more parks rather than fewer and that, in any case, parks were no place for free public baths. The *Times'* objection to locating baths in parks failed to move the city authorities, who were, however, impressed by the neighborhood opposition, and the Tompkins Square site was dropped. In June 1896 a new site was selected in a proposed new park, also on the Lower East Side. This bath, the Seward Park Bath, which did not open until 1904, was the first of four baths to be located in public parks.[24]

Once this decision was made, the question of municipal baths was quiescent for the remainder of 1896, but interest revived in early 1897 mainly as a result of the publication in book form of the Mayor's Committee official *Report on Public Baths and Comfort Stations*. This report, an important document in the municipal bath movement and the first major work on the subject to appear in this country, was mostly the work of William H. Tolman, the secretary of the committee. It was 249 pages, lavishly illustrated, and surveyed municipal baths in detail in Europe and the United States. The cost of publishing the report was raised by private subscription after the city government failed to provide the necessary funds. The report once again urged that the city build public baths: "It is needless to mention the imperative necessity of a sufficient number of free public baths in a great city like New York." The report further asserted that the operation of public baths was "clearly a municipal function."[25]

The Mayor's Committee *Report* prompted favorable editorial comment in the New York press and criticism of the Strong administration for its inaction. The *New York Daily Tribune* expressed hope that the report would "not be left to moulder among the musty documents of things talked about" and chided the city for going no further in the building of public baths than picking out a "site on a small park yet to be created." The *New York Times* also editorialized that there was "an urgent need of cheap and attractive public facilities for bathing" in New York City and once again urged the Strong administration to act quickly.[26]

In spite of the revival of interest in public baths, further delay ensued as confusion developed over the issue of whether the Public Bath Law of 1896 actually required that baths be located in public parks. The mayor and his committee thought it did, but Simon Baruch, supported by the press and his fellow physicians in the New York Academy of Medicine, insisted that baths could be located on sites other than parks. It is not clear whether Baruch and his supporters were able to convince Mayor Strong of the correctness of their interpretation, but a site at 326 Rivington Street, where the city owned the land, was selected for New York City's first municipal bath. In December 1897, two and one-half years after the passage of the mandatory bath law of 1895, ground was broken at this site. The Rivington Street Bath, which did not open until March 23, 1901, cost $95,691 and had 91 showers and 10 bathtubs. In building such a large bath, the city was following the recommendation of the Mayor's Committee rather than that of Baruch and the New York press, which favored smaller baths.[27]

In 1897 New York City's reformers organized for the mayoral election of that year. Mayor Strong had declined to run for another term, and the coalition of reformers who had formed the Committee of Seventy had disintegrated. Although Strong had achieved success in reforming the police department, the sanitation department, and the public school system, questions of patronage, of economy and efficiency versus increased expenditures for education and welfare, and conflict over Sunday closing laws combined to destroy the coalition which had elected him. In its place a narrower group of reformers, mainly Protestant and Jewish philanthropists, charity workers, and moral reformers, organized the Citizens' Union under the leadership of R. Fulton Cutting. Cutting, a patrician descendant of Robert Livingston and Robert Fulton and a leading New York financier and philanthropist, was active in the cause of municipal baths as president of the AICP from 1892 to 1921, president of the Citizens' Union from 1897 to 1909, and one of the founders of the Bureau of Municipal Research. All these organizations played an important role in New York's municipal bath movement. It is no surprise then that the Citizens' Union's first publication was a pamphlet entitled *Public Baths and Lavatories,* which urged the construction of more municipal baths.[28]

The mayoral election of 1897 was a crucial one both because the mayor would serve for four years instead of two and because he would be the mayor of Greater New York, as a result of the proposed consolidation of

New York City and the surrounding areas, including the city of Brooklyn, into one giant city. The reformers selected as their candidate Seth Low, former mayor of Brooklyn and president of Columbia University. Republicans, however, put forth their own candidate, General Benjamin F. Tracy, a close friend of the Republican boss, Thomas Platt. The Tammany Democrats ran Judge Robert Van Wyck on the slogan "To hell with reform." With Republican and reform votes divided, the election of Van Wyck was a foregone conclusion.[29]

The loss of reform influence apparently disheartened the bath advocates temporarily, for during the first eighteen months of Van Wyck's administration there was little activity, except for a mass meeting of Lower East Side residents at the University Settlement who demanded public baths. By the middle of 1899, however, both the *New York Daily Tribune* and Simon Baruch, in a letter to that newspaper, praised the efforts of the Strong administration to comply with the mandatory bath law of 1895 and deplored the failure of the Van Wyck administration to build more municipal baths.[30]

Finally, in June 1899, the Van Wyck administration moved to placate New York's municipal bath advocates by requesting approval from the board of estimate of a bond issue of $300,000 for municipal baths to be located in all five boroughs of the city. But no subsequent action was taken, apparently because of opposition from the city controller, who stated later that he felt the city had too many other expenses and was dangerously near the debt limit.[31]

From this point in 1899 until the Rivington Street Bath opened in March 1901, no further progress was made by the municipal bath movement in New York City. In 1900, after more than a decade of agitation and a great deal of ostensible progress, the city still did not have a single year-round municipal bath.

Several factors account for this lack of actual accomplishment. In the early 1890s the Tammany-controlled mayoral administrations of Hugh J. Grant and Thomas F. Gilroy showed no interest at all in the bath movement. Despite the passage of the permissive bath law no move was made by the city administrations to implement it. They explained their reluctance in terms of lack of public interest, which probably was an important factor. At no time during this period was there much genuine popular demand for municipal baths. Reformers and the local press were the main supporters of public baths.

The election of the reform mayor William L. Strong, who supported public baths and the passage of the mandatory public bath law of 1895, should have brought prompt success for New York's municipal bath movement, but for various reasons it did not. Confusion over whether the public bath law of 1896 required that baths be located in parks caused delay, as did the ongoing move toward the creation of Greater New York, which became reality on January 1, 1898. This impending change gave the Strong administration a sense of impermanence and insecurity and made it unwilling to commit itself to change in many areas. The return of Tammany control in 1898 caused further delay as Tammany was still not interested in the subject and made only a token move to plan for further baths, which achieved no results.[32]

It was not only the political situation, however, that contributed to the comparative failure of the movement for public baths. The leaders of the movement were also responsible. They were not unified and never organized as a group to put effective pressure on the municipal authorities. Their activities throughout most of this period were sporadic rather than sustained. The activities of Goodwin Brown in Albany, which resulted in the passage of the laws of 1892 and 1895, were not coordinated with those of the city bath reformers, and he, in fact, jealously stated that he was solely responsible for these laws. Although Simon Baruch worked with the AICP in the building of the People's Baths and attempted to influence the Tammany administrations, he was not a member of either the Committee of Seventy's Sub-Committee on Baths and Lavatories or of the Mayor's Committee and thus did not lend his influence to their efforts.

From 1887 to 1900 the political situation in New York City, confusion during the administration of its one reform mayor, public indifference, and the disunity of the bath reformers themselves all combined to produce only very modest results in the municipal bath movement.

## Success and Misgivings, 1901–1915

The fourteen years following the opening of the Rivington Street Bath in March 1901 were in complete contrast to the previous decade, for now the bath advocates, under the leadership of the AICP, at last achieved resounding success. The city heeded their demands and built sixteen more public baths in Manhattan, seven in Brooklyn, and one each in the

Bronx and Queens. Only rural Staten Island did not get a public bath. Shower baths were also set up in twenty-six public schools. During this period, the AICP also assumed a watchdog role by attempting to ensure that the baths were well patronized and economically and efficiently operated.

Even before the Rivington Street Bath was opened, the AICP criticized the Van Wyck administration for extravagance. Commissioner Henry S. Kearny of the Department of Public Buildings, Lighting and Supplies, under whose jurisdiction the new bathhouse fell, had requested the sum of $51,947.50 for the first year's operation of the bath, and $35,000 had been appropriated. The AICP, in a letter to the mayor, objected and stated:

It is the belief of the Board of Managers of this Association, founded upon eight years' practical knowledge of the matter, that the expenditure of any such sum as $35,000 for one year's maintenance of the Free Public Bath in Rivington Street, is unnecessary, unwarranted, and prejudicial to progress in extending the public bath system.

They further offered to operate the bath for the first year for $17,500.[33]

This controversy was well publicized and debated in the press. Kearny defended himself by noting that the bath was much larger than the People's Baths and was required to be open sixteen hours per day and that city employees worked only eight hours per day while AICP employees could work twelve. The AICP responded by renewing their $17,500 offer. An editorial in the *New York Daily Tribune* commented that the difference between the AICP figures and Kearny's figures represented "the margin of official waste in the Tammany method of conducting a public enterprise as compared with the cost of doing the same work under the management of plain businessmen." In the end Kearny was forced to reduce his estimate of the amount necessary to maintain and operate the bath to $24,272. He pledged that he would try "to keep the expenditures within this estimate and can assure you that I will hold myself responsible for any extravagance or wanton expenditure of money."[34]

The official opening of the Rivington Street Bath in March 1901, although it occurred without fanfare, received ample coverage in the press in both favorable editorials and feature stories. The *New York Daily Tribune* reported that the new bath had "been received with joy by the men, women and children of the overcrowded district of the East Side." The strongest press campaign for more municipal baths came in July 1901, when the *Evening Post* published a three-part series of feature articles on its front pages. Appealing to civic pride, the *Post* pointed out how far New York City lagged behind the cities of Europe and other American cities in the building of public baths. It attributed the delay to Tammany Hall and asked why "Tammany ever anxious to undertake building jobs and to compass public works which appeal ostentatiously to the people" had shown so little interest in public baths. Citing the great need for public baths and the necessity of educating the poor on the importance of regular bathing, the articles asserted that it was the city's duty to provide public baths. Editorially, the *Post* urged economy: "What New York needs is a large number of small cheap baths, scattered throughout the crowded districts, not on such a lavish scale as the one bathhouse in Rivington Street."[35]

In the face of these demands and the upcoming mayoral election in November 1901, the Van Wyck administration took action. First, the president of the board of education requested an appropriation of $30,000 for shower baths to be located in the basements of ten public schools, stating that he considered "the school bath system as important as the system of school libraries." Then Commissioner Kearny recommended that five new baths be built in Manhattan, three in Brooklyn, and one each in the Bronx, Queens, and Staten Island at a cost of $33,000 each, these new facilities to be smaller and less costly than the first bath.[36]

The AICP was quick to criticize this recommendation. Its president, R. Fulton Cutting, and its general agent, Frank Tucker, claimed that the city had underestimated the cost of land and building. Inexpensive baths of this kind, they said, would not stand up to the wear and tear of constant use and would not provide enough light and ventilation. At the October board of estimate meeting, a resolution was introduced calling for a bond issue of $350,000 to provide for eleven free baths. The board, however, referred the matter to the city controller and no further action was taken at that time.[37]

It seems obvious that the flurry of activity regarding the question of municipal baths on the part of the Tammany administration of Mayor Van Wyck was a response to the concentrated newspaper campaign for baths in the summer of 1901. More than likely it was also in preparation for the approaching mayoral election of November 1901. In this campaign both Tammany and the reform and Republican forces, now united behind the candidacy of Seth Low, came out for the establishment of more free baths in New York City.

Seth Low won the mayoral election of 1901 and proved to be an effective, if not especially popular, reform mayor. A former businessman, two-term mayor of Brooklyn before the Greater New York consolidation, and former president of Columbia University, Low provided the city with an honest and progressive government which strictly enforced existing laws and enacted many reforms.[38]

The bath reformers were not slow in presenting their case to the Low administration. In February 1902, the Public Bath Committee of the AICP, chaired by John Seely Ward, Jr., and including among its members Eugene Delano, former president of the board of trustees of the Public Baths Association of Philadelphia, sent a report to Manhattan's borough president, Jacob A. Cantor, who was now charged with responsibility for the existing bath. This detailed report began by reviewing the success of the People's Baths and the Rivington Street Bath, as well as municipal baths in other cities, such as Philadelphia, Baltimore, and Boston. It asserted that public baths should be located in the centers of densely populated districts and "should look clean, feel warm, smell sweet, have a generous supply of hot water and be conducted in a quiet, orderly way." The report recommended that the city construct sixteen more bathhouses in Manhattan to attain an adequate municipal bath system in the borough, as well as suggesting sites and including architect's plans for these new baths. In spite of the feeling on the part of many bath advocates that future baths should be smaller and less expensive than the Rivington Street Bath, the AICP's recommendations were for the larger, more expensive type of bath, which, it maintained, would be more economical to build (cost less per shower compartment) and to maintain. The city followed these recommendations for larger baths and located future Manhattan baths, as a rule, in the vicinity of the sites suggested in this report (see table 3.1).[39]

The AICP report and recommendations were publicized by the press, and for the first time the people as well as city officials supported the municipal bath reformers in New York. Borough President Cantor expressed his approval of the report and promised to have a measure introduced at the next meeting of the board of aldermen appropriating $300,000 for municipal baths.[40]

Table 3.1.   Municipal Baths of New York City, 1915[a]

| Bath | Year of Opening | Cost of Construction | Cost of Land | Total Cost |
|---|---|---|---|---|
| *Manhattan* | | | | |
| 326 Rivington St. | 1901 | $95,691 | City owned | $95,691 |
| 327 West 41st St. | 1904 | 101,550 | $33,750 | 135,300 |
| 133 Allen St. | 1905 | 92,935 | 34,805 | 127,740 |
| 538 East 11th St. | 1905 | 102,989 | 22,000 | 124,989 |
| 243 East 109th St. | 1905 | 110,953 | 19,000 | 129,953 |
| 232 West 60th St. | 1906 | 126,550 | 12,750 | 139,300 |
| 523 East 76th St. | 1906 | 104,844 | 11,000 | 115,844 |
| 83 Carmine St. | 1908 | 132,954 | 77,190 | 210,144 |
| 23rd St. and Ave. A | 1908 | 259,432 | City owned | 259,432 |
| 100 Cherry St. | 1909 | 150,985 | 54,363 | 205,348 |
| 5 Rutgers Pl. | 1909 | 184,195 | 80,000 | 264,195 |
| 342 East 54th St. | 1911 | 244,800 | 72,500 | 317,300 |
| 407 West 28th St. | 1914 | 170,000 | 56,000 | 226,000 |
| *Brooklyn* | | | | |
| Hicks St. | 1903 | 58,043 | 3,750 | 61,793 |
| Pitkin Ave. | 1903 | 84,456 | 4,000 | 88,456 |
| Montrose Ave. | b | 95,792 | 2,500 | 96,042 |
| Huron St. | b | 97,924 | 5,800 | 103,724 |
| Duffield St. | b | 97,493 | 13,500 | 110,993 |
| Wilson Ave. | b | b | b | b |
| *Bronx* | | | | |
| 156th St. and Elton Ave. | 1909 | b | b | b |

[a]New York City, *Annual Report of the Business and Transactions of the President of the Borough of Manhattan, City of New York for the Year Ending December 31, 1915,* excerpt from table A. The baths in public parks were located at Seward Park, 138th St. and 5th Ave., 52nd St. and 11th Ave., and 111th St. and 1st Ave. (William Paul Gerhard, *Modern Baths,* 107; Stanley H. Howe, *History, Condition and Needs of Public Baths in Manhattan*).

[b]Figures unavailable. The location and cost of the bath located in Queens are also unavailable.

Within three weeks, the Citizens' Union sponsored a mass meeting on public baths held in Pacific Hall on the Lower East Side. The speakers included R. Fulton Cutting, president of both the AICP and the Citizens' Union, who spoke on the hygienic virtues of frequent baths, and W. H. Baldwin, Jr., the president of the Long Island Railroad, who spoke on the historic baths of Rome. The principal speaker was Charles Sprague-Smith, who, with Cutting and others, was a founder of the People's Institute, which offered a forum for adult education on the major issues of the day. Sprague-Smith urged the fulfillment of the Low administration's campaign promises to establish "public baths open all year through" and climaxed his speech with the peroration, "Thus, with physical and mental health renewed through cleansed bodies, the people will more intelligently consider the great problem of democracy—which is theirs to solve." The meeting concluded with the adoption of a resolution requesting the city to provide a public bathhouse in the vicinity of the block bounded by Chrystie, Forsyth, Bayard, and Canal streets, one of the sites suggested by the AICP report. In midtown Manhattan, about three hundred persons attended a West Side Neighborhood House meeting urging the city to establish a municipal bath in their neighborhood (West 50th Street).[41]

In Brooklyn, both the Citizens' Union and the Women's Municipal League held public meetings urging board of estimate approval of municipal baths, and the *Brooklyn Daily Eagle* added its editorial voice to the agitation: "We shall never have a beautiful city till we have a clean city, and the city will never be clean when masses of its inhabitants are dirty." It urged the city to "build baths, big ones, handsome ones, and in every crowded quarter of the town."[42]

In the face of mounting demands, the Board of Estimate and Apportionment in June 1902 approved an appropriation of $480,000 for public baths, an appropriation which had already been approved by the board of aldermen by a vote of sixty-two to one. Three baths were to be provided for Manhattan and two for Brooklyn. Sparked by the election of reformer Seth Low and by the publication of the AICP report, the bath reformers had achieved a substantial victory. Moreover, they had now succeeded in arousing public opinion in favor of municipal baths. It cannot be ascertained how many of the bath advocates who attended the meetings described above would become bath users, but it seems that at least some slum dwellers were actively in favor of municipal baths, especially in Manhattan. In Brooklyn, most of the support came from middle class reformers.[43]

During the remainder of 1902, plans moved forward quickly for the five baths for which appropriations had been made. Sites were chosen by the borough presidents of Manhattan and Brooklyn, and architects' plans were approved by the Municipal Art Commission. The baths were to be located on 50 by 100-foot lots and each was to contain about 100 shower baths with connecting dressing rooms and a few tubs. They were to be imposing in appearance with an architectural style recalling ancient Roman public baths with classical pilasters, columns, arches, and cornices. Substantial materials were to be used throughout; one bath, for example, was to be constructed with brick, terra cotta, stone marble, and copper, and the front was to consist of "ornamental iron work, brick, white Italian marble and granite."[44]

While plans for the new bathhouse proceeded, the New York press continued to publicize the progress of the bath movement in 1902. In feature articles it not only reported the selection of sites and approval of architect's plans but also discussed the virtues of the Rivington Street Bath. Editorially, the press cited the necessity for municipal baths, congratulated the Low administration for its great progress, and urged the city to build more baths so that every slum dweller would have access to them.[45]

Although the city government was now assuming responsibility, private philanthropy did not abandon the public bath movement. In June 1902, Elizabeth Milbank Anderson announced that she would donate a public bath, to be built on a 50 by 98-foot lot on East 38th Street, to the AICP. Anderson was heiress to one of the founders of the Borden Condensed Milk Company and was a leading New York philanthropist. During her lifetime she donated approximately $5 million to various institutions, with Barnard College as the chief beneficiary. The bath which she donated, known as the Milbank Memorial Bath, opened in January 1904. A large and imposing facility, it cost $140,000 to build and could accommodate 3,000 bathers daily. In 1914, after a canvass of the neighborhood, the AICP established a wet-wash laundry at the Milbank bath.[46]

The Low administration continued its interest in municipal baths, and in 1903 appropriations were approved and sites selected for five additional baths in Manhattan. The largest and finest of these was the neo-

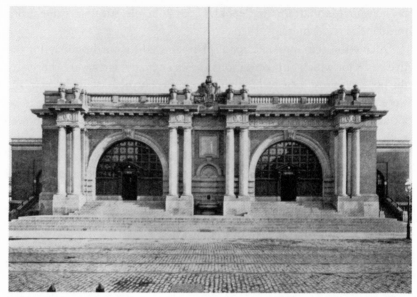

Monumental Neo-Roman East 23rd Street Public Bath, New York City, 1908; Arnold W. Brunner and William Martin Aiken, architects. Source: Museum of the City of New York.

Roman East 23rd Street Bath, which was to include a swimming pool and would cost $225,000. This bath, now housing indoor and outdoor swimming pools and renamed the Asser Levy Bath, has since been designated an official landmark by the Landmarks Preservation Commission. After years of neglect, it underwent an $8 million restoration and reopened in 1990.[47]

In 1903, control of the city government reverted to Tammany, as the Democrats elected George B. McClellan over the incumbent Low, again nominated by the reformers. In this election both candidates had come out strongly for expanding the municipal bath system, but it remained to be seen if Tammany, so long indifferent to the cause of public baths, would fulfill its preelection promises.[48]

By now, however, Tammany, under the more enlightened and progressive rule of boss Charles Francis Murphy, seemed to have wholeheartedly endorsed the cause of municipal baths, for in May 1904 the sum of $1,050,000 was appropriated by the Board of Estimate and Apportionment for eight additional baths: four to be located in Manhattan, three in Brooklyn, and one in the Bronx. With the building of these baths, New York's municipal bath system was nearly complete. Construction closely followed the suggestions of the AICP report of 1902. The bathhouses were large, elaborate, and imposing edifices which eventually cost the city almost $4 million to build.[49]

Table 3.1 shows that the municipal baths grew increasingly costly; the least expensive bath was the first one built. The baths also grew more elaborate, and by 1915, six of them were equipped with indoor swimming pools. The West 28th Street Bath, for example, in addition to showers and an indoor swimming pool, had public laundry facilities, a gymnasium with an indoor track, and a roof garden and playground. Five other baths also had gymnasiums. Very likely the growing emphasis on the recreational as opposed to the cleanliness function of the public baths accounts for more public enthusiasm and Tammany support.[50]

New York City's public baths were located mostly in slum neighborhoods and customarily served one immigrant group, although no neighborhoods were completely homogeneous (see map 1). In Manhattan, baths on Rivington Street, Rutgers Place, and in Seward Park served the Jewish Lower East Side. Irish immigrants and their children could bathe in the bathhouses on Cherry Street on the Lower East Side, West 28th Street in Chelsea, East 23rd Street in the Gashouse District, and West 60th Street in Hell's Kitchen. The proximity of the West 60th Street Bath to the African-American neighborhood called San Juan Hill caused clashes between Irish and black youths who used the bath. Baths were located in Little Italys at Carmine Street in Greenwich Village and East 109th and East 111th streets in Italian Harlem. The East 76th Street Bath was in Little Bohemia, a Czech and Hungarian neighborhood within Yorkville, a larger German neighborhood. The East 54th Street Bath accommodated a largely poor Irish clientele when it opened in 1911, but this bath was located near Beekman and Sutton places, which became fashionable addresses in the 1920s. The juxtaposition of slums and luxury apartment houses here is supposed to have inspired Sidney Kingsley's 1930s play *Dead End*, although the Dead End kids bathed in the East River rather than the nearby public bath, which had a swimming pool. The 138th Street Bath served African Americans in Harlem, and the East 11th Street Bath was in the heart of the old German district.[51]

New York City also situated two public baths in vice and entertainment districts. The Allen Street Bath was in a red light district on the

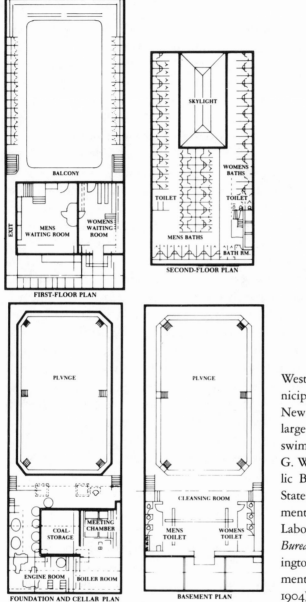

West 60th Street Municipal Bath, New York, New York. Floor plan, large bathhouse with swimming pool. Source: G. W. W. Hanger, "Public Baths in the United States," U.S. Department of Commerce and Labor, *Bulletin of the Bureau of Labor* 9 (Washington, D.C., Government Printing Office, 1904), Plate 157.

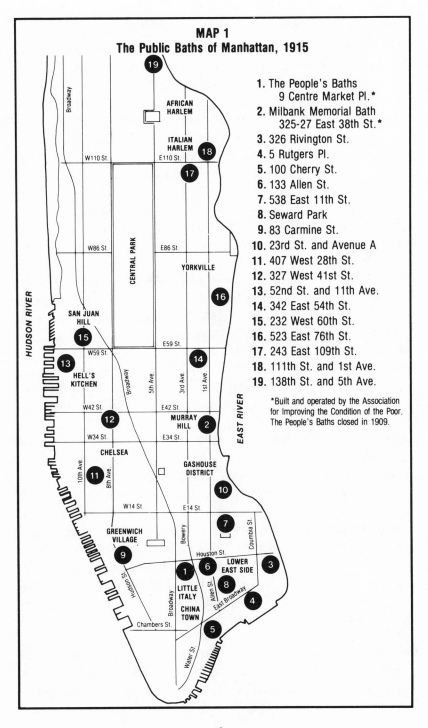

**MAP 1**
**The Public Baths of Manhattan, 1915**

1. The People's Baths
   9 Centre Market Pl.*
2. Milbank Memorial Bath
   325-27 East 38th St.*
3. 326 Rivington St.
4. 5 Rutgers Pl.
5. 100 Cherry St.
6. 133 Allen St.
7. 538 East 11th St.
8. Seward Park
9. 83 Carmine St.
10. 23rd St. and Avenue A
11. 407 West 28th St.
12. 327 West 41st St.
13. 52nd St. and 11th Ave.
14. 342 East 54th St.
15. 232 West 60th St.
16. 523 East 76th St.
17. 243 East 109th St.
18. 111th St. and 1st Ave.
19. 138th St. and 5th Ave.

*Built and operated by the Association
for Improving the Condition of the Poor.
The People's Baths closed in 1909.

Lower East Side, and the West 41st Street Bath was in the Tenderloin near Times Square. Mostly likely these baths were meant to serve a transient population as well as the residents of the area.[52]

Despite their success in achieving an elaborate system of municipal baths in New York City, the bath advocates did not rest on their laurels. From 1905 to 1915 they pressed increasingly hard for improvements in the public bath system. Their chief criticisms of the public baths were that the patronage did "not begin to tax their capacity" and that they were extravagant in construction and inefficient in their management. Bath reformers, like other progressive reformers of this era, became obsessed with economy and efficiency. The AICP led the attack in its 1905 annual report, which criticized the administration of the bath system on several counts. It noted the delay in completion of new baths as contractors repeatedly violated the time limits of their contracts. It asserted that the city government was spending large sums of money "filtering water for bathing purposes, which the bathers use for drinking purposes in their own homes unfiltered." The AICP also found payroll and repair accounts unnecessarily high and maintained that the city was not receiving a fair return for money expended. There is no evidence that the municipal government made any response to these criticisms.[53]

The AICP not only criticized the municipal bath system but took steps to increase the patronage of the baths, as in the case of the East 109th Street Bath in the Italian section of Harlem. Built at a cost of over $129,000, this bath was equipped with 122 showers, seven tubs, marble partitions and floors, and hot and cold filtered water. Despite the bath's attractiveness, only 150 persons patronized it during the first week after its opening in March 1905. The AICP then sent an agent to the neighborhood to publicize the new bath. He visited stores, shops, and factories, and addressed classes at the local public and parochial schools. He and the teachers took groups of children to the bath and sent them home with letters printed in Italian and addressed to their parents regarding the bath. During the fourth week after the opening, patronage increased to 4,712 and the publicity campaign was deemed a success.[54]

Robert E. Todd of the Bureau of Municipal Research also criticized the public baths on the grounds of underutilization. In two articles which appeared in the magazine *Charities* and *The Survey* in 1907 and 1910, Todd noted that during the cooler months the baths were used at only 4–25 percent of capacity, a utilization "disproportionate to the extravagant expense under which the municipal baths are maintained." This lack of patronage, Todd felt, was due to the fact that the baths had "been constructed on a social base that [was] narrow and largely false, the purpose having been to meet a 'felt want' in the crowded tenement districts." Todd believed that this "felt want" did not exist except in the heat of summer and that the only way to increase public use of the municipal baths was to include swimming pools and gymnasiums, which would attract patrons, especially children and young persons, who would be educated in the habit of bathing regularly. This educational purpose was what Todd considered, very perceptively, to be the most important function of the municipal baths.[55] Actually the New York City government recognized this fact, and most baths built after 1904 contained a swimming pool and some also had a gymnasium.

In 1913 the AICP once again urged the city to improve the municipal bath system. Observing that the capacity of the municipal baths was 61,965 persons daily and that in 1911 the average daily attendance had been only 9,813, it recommended that the city immediately begin a campaign of popularization of the baths to make them more widely known and generally attractive. The AICP also recommended the formation of a Bureau of Public Baths with a superintendent at its head rather than supervision by the individual borough presidents. The association urged that all new baths include public laundries as part of their facilities, that public school baths be open during evening hours, and that all public baths be open all day Sunday. It felt that the baths should be permitted to close early in the winter months when patronage was low, a change which would have required amendment of the Bath Law of 1895. Finally, although the AICP criticized the municipal government for its failure to attract patrons to the baths, it urged the city to build additional small baths in the tenement districts. Once again the municipal government did not respond to any of these criticisms or implement any of the recommendations.[56]

This list of recommendations from the AICP appears to have been the last action taken by the bath reformers to improve the baths of New York City. Although the press reported the AICP's recommendations, it did not support them editorially, and there seems to have been no reaction on the part of the public. The opening of the West 28th Street Bath in 1914 brought to a close the period of construction of New York's municipal system, except for the building in the late 1920s of an additional bath on West 134th Street to serve Harlem, where African Americans had moved in large numbers during and after World War I.[57]

The major concern of the bath reformers, once an adequate system of baths was under construction, was the fact that the baths were not patronized to anywhere near their capacity except on the hottest summer days. In Manhattan, for example, patronage for 1906, when seven baths were open, amounted to 3,162,811; in 1915, the first year that all the municipal baths were in operation, it was 7,385,496; in 1920 it was 7,500,056; and in 1933 it was 6,811,605. When it is considered that the actual capacity of Manhattan's baths was over 20 million per year the patronage seems very low indeed. Meanwhile the cost of maintaining the bath system steadily increased: for example, from $254,040 for 1913 to $362,919 in 1919 in Manhattan.[58]

The underutilization of New York's municipal baths except on the hottest summer days can be explained partly by the fact that, although a need for public baths existed in view of the lack of bath facilities in slum tenement dwellings, this need was not felt by the majority of the tenement house population for whom the baths were intended. Tenement house dwellers apparently did not have the habit of bathing regularly year-round or preferred the limited facilities of their own homes. The increased patronage of the baths in the summer and the continuing popularity of the floating baths can be explained by the fact that people were sweatier and dirtier in the summer and felt more need for a complete bath. No doubt they also used the baths as a means of cooling off or as recreation.

Another reason for the low patronage of the baths was the increasing number of tenements equipped with bathing facilities. Although the Tenement House Law of 1901 did not require that each new apartment have a bathtub, it did require that each apartment have a private toilet, and most new tenements included a private bathtub as well. A consequence of this new construction was that the owners of many older buildings were forced to add separate bathing and toilet facilities or risk having their tenants move. In 1906 Superintendent of the People's Baths R. E. Taylor explained their declining patronage to the AICP: "Landlords are putting tubs—bath tubs—in all new flats down this way and when they overhaul an old building. [*sic*] One place only two blocks from here there have been twenty-four bath-tubs installed during pass [*sic*] month." Perhaps if the bath system had been completed in the 1890s, before such housing reform was instituted, it might have been better patronized. Or, if the baths had not been so large and expensive, the amount of patronage that did exist would have been considered satisfactory.[59]

After 1915, the bath movement lost vigor, and those reformers who remained interested transferred their efforts to the American Association for Promoting Hygiene and Public Baths, a professional organization of bath reformers and administrators founded in 1912 with Simon Baruch as president. Most of New York's municipal baths were renovated in the 1930s by the Works Progress Administration and continued to operate during World War II. After the war, however, they were either demolished to make way for other structures, converted to other uses, or maintained by the city as public swimming pools and gymnasiums. Only one of Manhattan's baths, the Allen Street Bath, continued to serve its original purpose until New York's fiscal crisis of the 1970s forced its closing.[60]

# 4

## Patrician Mayors, Irish Bosses, and "Municipal Housekeepers": The Municipal Baths of Boston and Chicago

### The Municipal Baths of Boston

> The inauguration of winter bath-houses for the free use of the people is something of a novelty in any city in this country, and Boston has the proud distinction of being the pioneer in the work, which is sure to be an important consideration in the growing demand of the larger municipalities in the near future.

On October 15, 1898, the *Boston Herald* proudly reported the opening of Boston's first year-round municipal bathhouse, the Dover Street Bath. The opening ceremony was attended by more than 500 persons, with the Back Bay well represented, as well as a "large number of men and women who [were] identified with educational and sociological questions of the city." Mayor Josiah Quincy, the leader of Boston's public bath movement and the main speaker, proclaimed, "The opening of this bath marks the full recognition by the city of its duty to bring within the reach of all in winter as well as in summer, facilities for securing the physical cleanliness that bears such close relationship to social and moral well-being." This occasion marked the culmination of many years of effort by Boston sanitarians and social reformers to provide the poor with a means of attaining personal cleanliness.[1]

As we have seen, the massive Irish immigration of the 1840s and the overcrowding, lack of sanitation, and filth of the slums in which these immigrants lived, as well as economic depression and cholera epidemics, prompted the first demands for public baths. The Massachusetts Sanitary Commission in 1850 and a special joint committee of the board of aldermen and the common council in 1860 had urged that Boston provide bathing facilities for its poor, but the city had not responded to these recommendations. Beginning in 1866, however, the city had built fourteen floating baths and one beach bath, which were operated by the board of health during the summer months. These baths did not resolve the question of year-round cleanliness, but the Commonwealth of Massachusetts took a step in this direction in 1874, when it passed enabling legislation permitting any town to purchase or lease lands, erect public baths and washhouses, and raise or appropriate money for these purposes.[2]

It was not until the early 1890s, however, that any action was taken to implement the Massachusetts Bath Law. The need for year-round public baths was first publicized by Robert A. Woods, who became head resident of Andover House Settlement in Boston's South End in 1892. Believing that settlement-house workers ought to call attention to the needs of their neighborhoods, Woods and the residents of Andover House made regular trips to city hall to appeal to the city council for a public bath. The council listened to their requests but refused to appropriate the money.[3]

Woods, whom Arthur Mann has called "the philosopher and tactician of the university settlement," was born in Pittsburgh in 1865 of middle class, Scotch-Irish, rigidly Presbyterian parentage. He graduated from Amherst College in 1886 and then attended Andover Theological Seminary. Rather than entering the ministry, however, Woods was attracted to the idea of service through the social settlement movement. In 1891 he went to England to study Toynbee Hall so that a similar establishment could be set up in Boston under the auspices of Andover Theological Seminary, with Woods as its head.[4]

Woods' approach to municipal reform was realistic and pragmatic rather than doctrinaire and monistic. As Mann has noted, Woods scorned the reformers

who thought the millennium would come by throwing out the bosses and getting honest businessmen to run the city. . . . The question was not who ran the government but how it was run; the crucial municipal issue was to extend political functions to satisfy the needs of the poor, to give them baths, gymnasiums, sanitary tenements, parks, playgrounds, clean streets, industrial education.

Thus, municipal baths were only one aspect of Woods' campaign against urban poverty, but in Josiah Quincy, who was elected Boston's mayor in 1895, he found an ally in his realistic approach and in particular in his demand for baths.[5]

Josiah Quincy, a member of a patrician and public-spirited Boston family, was the third Mayor Quincy of Boston, for his father and great-grandfather had been mayor before him. Quincy was born in 1859 and was educated at Harvard College and Harvard Law School. He entered politics in 1884, when as a Democrat he campaigned for Cleveland against Blaine. In 1887–88 and 1890–91 Quincy served in the state house of representatives, where he was a member of the committee on cities and worked for the secret ballot law. He was chairman of the Democratic State Committee in 1891–92. In 1893 he was appointed assistant secretary of state by President Cleveland, a position from which he resigned to run for mayor of Boston.[6]

Raised in a tradition of social paternalism, inspired by the progress of the great cities of Europe in meeting the needs of their citizens, and influenced by his creative friendship with Robert Woods, Quincy, as mayor, determined to bring to Boston a panoply of social innovations including public baths (which were probably his favorite project), playgrounds, public gymnasiums, boys' summer camps, public concerts, and free lectures. Although Quincy is usually considered a reform mayor, he was supported in his election bid by boss Czar Martin Lomasney and worked with Boston's other bosses (Smiling Jim Donovan of the South End, Joseph Corbett and Patrick J. Kennedy of East Boston, John F. Fitzgerald of the North End, and other district leaders) through an informal group dubbed the Board of Strategy. He also cooperated with organized labor and with Boston's leading citizens, social reformers, and philanthropists, whom he involved in the municipal government by appointing them to unpaid commissions, departments, and ad hoc committees in a kind of "participatory bureaucracy." Quincy wrote of his vision of Boston as a community:

The duty of a city is to promote the civilization, in the fullest sense of the word, of all its citizens. No true civilization can exist without the provision of some reasonable opportunities for exercising the physical and mental faculties, of experiencing something of the variety and of the healthful pleasures of life, or feeling at least the degree of self-respect which personal cleanliness brings with it. The people of a city constitute a community, in all which that significant term implies; their interests are inextricably bound up together, and everything which promotes the well-being of a large part of the population benefits all.[7]

The municipal government of Boston in 1895 at the time of Quincy's election as mayor was unwieldy and in the hands of Irish bosses. The mayor had only moderate executive power, and most of his executive decisions had to be approved by the board of aldermen, which was composed of twelve members elected at large. The common council, the legislative branch, had 72 members elected by district. The real power in the municipal government was in the joint committees of the board of aldermen and the common council, of which there were 56 in 1895. In the same year the mayoral term was changed from one year to two. During his two terms as mayor, Quincy was able to link the diverging classes and interests of the citizens of Boston and for a brief time to make it, as Geoffrey Blodgett noted, "the cutting edge of urban reform in America."[8]

In his inaugural address on January 6, 1896, Quincy promised to take action on the issue of public baths:

The maintaining of public baths, open all the year seems to me to be a project for encouraging social and sanitary improvement by municipal action which promises large return for a comparatively small expenditure, and I am of [the] opinion that the experiment of establishing such a public bath in a suitable locality should be tried. I shall recommend such an appropriation to be provided for by loan.

On January 20, 1896, Quincy, probably following the precedent of New York City's reform mayor William L. Strong, announced the formation of the Mayor's Advisory Committee on Public Baths with Robert A. Woods as its chairman. The committee was to investigate the subject, estimate the cost, and recommend the best location for a public bath. It planned to visit New York City to confer with Mayor Strong's bath committee and inspect the People's Baths erected by the New York Association for Improving the Condition of the Poor.[9]

In addition to Woods, the membership of the Boston Bath Committee included Dr. Edward Mussey Hartwell, who was director of physical training in the public schools of Boston. Hartwell was born in 1850 in Exeter, New Hampshire, attended the Boston Latin School, and graduated from Amherst College in 1873. He received a Ph.D. from Johns Hopkins in 1881 and an M.D. from Miami Medical College in Cincinnati, Ohio, in 1882. Hartwell had taught in high school in the 1870s and was an instructor at Johns Hopkins from 1883 to 1891, when he became Boston's director of physical training. Hartwell was strongly in favor of public school baths and was also a prominent member of the National Municipal League, which was devoted to municipal reform. He wrote extensively on both municipal reform and public baths. In 1897 Mayor Quincy appointed him secretary of Boston's newly created Department of Municipal Statistics.[10]

Two women were also members of the mayor's advisory committee, Mary Morton Kehew and Laliah Pingree. Kehew, a very active social reformer, was president of the Women's Educational and Industrial Union, an organization founded to encourage both trade unionism among women workers and labor legislation beneficial to them. After the American Federation of Labor convention in Boston in 1903, Kehew organized the National Women's Trade Union League for the same purpose on a nationwide scale. Pingree was a former member of the Boston School Committee.[11]

Labor was also represented on the mayor's committee by two members, Edward J. Ryan, president of the Buildings' Trades Council, and Michael W. Myers, president of the Plumbers' Union. The seventh member was Edmund Billings, superintendent and treasurer of the Wells Memorial Institute, a social and educational club for young workingmen which provided them with space to meet, socialize, and hold informal classes and which housed a small library and a gymnasium with hot and cold water baths.[12]

In April 1896, the Mayor's Advisory Committee on Public Baths, after studying New York City's People's Baths, issued its preliminary report. The report recommended that the city build its first year-round bath in the vicinity of Dover Street and Harrison Avenue in the heart of the Irish slums of Boston's South End, that the bath be built on a 50 by 100-foot lot, contain at least 40 showers, and accommodate both men and women in absolutely distinct compartments with separate entrances and waiting rooms. It also stipulated that the bath be completely free to all and that at least $50,000—and preferably $65,000—should be appropriated for land and building. In May 1896, Mayor Quincy referred the committee's recommendations to the Joint Standing Committee on the Health Department of the board of aldermen and the city council.[13]

The Joint Standing Committee also visited New York City and was much impressed by the People's Baths. Its report to the board of aldermen and the city council, issued in June 1896, made recommendations similar to those of the Mayor's Advisory Committee. It proposed that $65,000 (to be raised by issuing 20-year bonds at 4 percent interest) be appropriated for a bath similar to the People's Baths and that it be located on a 50 by 100-foot lot. The committee also advised that a public lavatory not be connected to the bath and that public baths should not be located in public schools, although schools could maintain showers for the use of schoolchildren only. It urged that the municipal bath be placed under the jurisdiction of the board of health but made no recommendation on the matter of whether the baths should be free or subject to a small fee.[14]

The Joint Standing Committee's recommendations were the basis for a feature story in the *Boston Herald* which also contained photographs and descriptions of New York City's People's Baths. In addition, the *Herald* editorially urged the board of aldermen and the city council to take "prompt and favorable action" on the committee's recommendations, pointing out that other cities, including Chicago, Brookline, Yonkers, and Philadelphia, were well on the way to constructing their municipal bath systems. The *Herald* also recommended the building of school baths, noting that the school board was already conducting cooking and sewing classes and asking, "Is not cleanliness, rather than cooking, next to godliness?"[15]

During the summer of 1896, plans for Boston's first bathhouse advanced as the board of aldermen and the city council appropriated the $65,000 requested (a few months later the amount was increased to $86,000). Land was purchased at 249 Dover Street near the recommended site for $14,150, and Peabody and Stearns were chosen as architects. In November the architectural plans—which called for a 43 by 110-foot, two-story bathhouse with 50 showers (17 of them for women)—were approved and construction began.[16]

Controversy did arise during this time, however, over the provision of baths in the public schools. This involved the question not only of whether baths should be located in the public schools but, if so, whether they should exist for the exclusive use of schoolchildren or be opened to the general public after school hours. Hartwell had suggested that 28 shower baths be included in the plans for two new school buildings to be constructed in the near future. The school board was divided on the issue and school baths were rejected outright by the Schoolhouse Committee, which was in charge of school buildings. In October 1896, the controversy was resolved, however, when the Joint Committee on Hygiene of the board of aldermen and the city council reported favorably on school baths, and such baths were included in the two new school buildings. These baths, however, were used exclusively by schoolchildren until 1906, when they were opened in the evening to the general public under the supervision of the Baths Department.[17]

Another controversy arose over the question of whether the baths should be free. Those who favored a fee felt that the baths should not be a charity. Others argued, in Mayor Quincy's words, that "free baths would not pauperize the people any more than free textbooks and free public schools." The *Boston Herald* agreed with Quincy, asserting that free baths would be more democratic, that all citizens were indirectly or directly taxpayers and therefore joint owners of the bath, and that at any rate parks and libraries were free already. In the end it was decided that Boston's baths would be free, for "it was felt that the charge of even one cent might keep away the very people who most needed bathing." There was a fee of one cent each for soap and towel, however.[18]

While Boston's first municipal bathhouse was being constructed, Mayor Quincy, with the approval of the board of aldermen, created a Department of Baths, headed by an unsalaried Bath Commission of seven Boston citizens appointed by the mayor for one- to five-year terms. The secretary of the Bath Commission was also the superintendent of baths and a paid official. In addition to having jurisdiction over the new Dover Street Bath, the commission operated Boston's 14 floating baths, 2 swimming pools, its natural beach baths, public comfort stations, and a combined gymnasium and bath in East Boston donated to the city by Mrs. Daniel Ahl in 1897. The chairman of the Bath Commission was Thomas J. Lane, an Irish Catholic leader from East Boston who was active in community improvement efforts there. Of the original Mayor's Advisory Committee on Public Baths, only Robert A. Woods was a member of the Bath Commission. Other members were two physicians, John Duff and Henry Ehrlich; two women, Mrs. Lawrence Logan and Mrs. Jacob Hecht; and Leonard D. Ahl. As has been noted, bath reformers in general advocated the supervision of public bath systems by this type of commission.[19]

The formal opening of the Dover Street Bath took place on October 14, 1898, with Thomas J. Lane presiding and Mayor Quincy as the main speaker. Quincy declared with civic pride that "if a few American cities have been a few years ahead of us, we can truthfully claim that Boston now possesses the finest and most modern public bathing establishment upon this continent." This bath, which cost approximately $86,000 to build, was most certainly a monumental and luxurious municipal bath. It was 43 feet wide, 110 feet deep, and three stories high. The facade was granite on the first story and gray mottled brick with limestone trimming on the upper stories and was surmounted by an ornamental cornice of galvanized iron. There were two entrances and two waiting rooms, one for men and one for women. The waiting rooms had terrazzo mosaic floors and Knoxville marble walls, and marble staircases led to the baths on the second floor. The men's section had 30 showers and 3 bathtubs and the women's section 11 showers and 6 tubs. Each shower consisted of a dressing alcove with a seat and a bathing compartment. The partitions were marble, as was the floor in the bathing section. The third floor was devoted to janitor's and matron's quarters, and the basement contained a laundry for washing towels at which family laundry could also be done at moderate cost. The opening of the Dover Street Bath prompted the *Boston Herald* to urge in an editorial that permanent baths be established in every part of the city where needed (although it did not specify any exact locations) and to commend Mayor Quincy for the progress made in that direction.[20]

The Dover Street Bath, however, proved to be Boston's last structure built for the primary purpose of providing baths for those without such facilities in their homes. After 1899, municipal bath facilities were combined with gymnasiums, and the emphasis shifted slowly from cleanliness to physical fitness and recreation. From 1899 to 1902 four combined baths and gymnasiums were added to Boston's bath system. Typical of these was the Ward 13 Gymnasium and Bath, which had on its first floor a gymnasium and locker and dressing space for men and on its second floor locker and dressing space for women and 20 shower baths. Regular programs of physical examinations, exercises, and games were arranged and supervised by the Baths Department, which also arranged for swimming lessons at the floating baths, beaches, and swimming pools.[21]

Several factors probably account for this shift in emphasis from cleanliness to recreation. By 1898 Mayor Quincy saw a close connection between bathing and recreation: "It is . . . impossible to draw any line between the maintenance of an out-door bathing place in summer and an indoor bath in winter, or between a shower bath and a tub bath, serving only the purpose of promoting cleanliness, and the swimming-pool which answers the further purpose of affording facilities for exercise and recreation." Quincy felt that ideally the municipality would furnish for each local group of 20,000 or 25,000 people, "divided upon lines which are carefully drawn in reference to social conditions and affiliations," a bathing establishment (including showers, tubs, and swimming pool), gymnasium, and playground. The Bath Commission was also enthusiastic in its support of combined gymnasiums and baths. It claimed very optimistically and unrealistically in its 1902–03 *Annual Report:*

As to the general public benefit accruing from the work of the department, we were able to show a year ago from the report of the Institutions Registration Department that there had been a marked decrease in juvenile arrests during the past ten years, and we believe that the work of the Bath Department had been the greatest single agency in effecting this vital improvement in public morals. We believe also, that in due time it will become clear that the baths and gymnasia are serving distinctly to lower the disease rate and the death rate of the city.

Economy also played a role, for combined baths and gymnasiums generally were less expensive than the Dover Street Bath, and one criticism of the Quincy administration was that his social reforms brought an increase in municipal indebtedness and produced an "insolvent utopia." As was the case in New York City, after the turn of the century tenement-house reform required builders to install a toilet in each new apartment; most builders installed a bathtub as well, thus decreasing the need for public baths.[22]

During Mayor Quincy's second term, the Yankee-Irish coalition which had been the basis of his power began to disintegrate. His attempts to increase and concentrate executive authority and rationalize operations of the city government were thwarted by Martin Lomasney and opposed by other Irish bosses. Structural reformers were also dismayed by the increase in the city's indebtedness rising out of his social reform programs, for as John Koren has noted, his "administration of four years was assuredly progressive but also expensive." For these reasons he was not nominated for a third term as mayor.[23]

Quincy's first two successors, Republican Thomas N. Hart (1900–02) and Democrat Patrick Collins (1902–05), were fiscal conservatives who felt that Quincy had spent too much on social reforms. Collins criticized "benevolent socialism," opposed city borrowing, reduced debt levels, and vetoed many spending ideas, including a 1902 appropriations bill that would have provided for additional gymnasiums and baths.[24]

Yet, despite these mayors' lack of interest, Boston continued to build municipal baths and gymnasiums, if more slowly than bath advocates would have hoped. Under Mayor Hart four combined baths and gymnasiums were opened, although planning for these had commenced during the Quincy years. Also during his term in 1901 construction was begun on the large and elaborate Cabot Street Bath and Gymnasium in the Irish Roxbury section, but its opening was delayed until 1905 due to lack of appropriations. This bath, which cost approximately $100,000 to build and equip, had, in addition to approximately 50 showers, a swimming pool and a "large, finely equipped gymnasium."[25]

Boston's bath movement, however, was enthusiastically supported by Mayor John F. Fitzgerald, the first of Boston's Irish bosses to achieve the mayoralty and President John F. Kennedy's grandfather. During his first term, 1906–07, plans were completed for the construction of seven municipal buildings to be located in the slum wards of Boston to serve various ethnic groups. These buildings generally housed municipal offices, a public hall, a branch of the public library with a reading room, a gymnasium, swimming pool, and shower baths. During his second term, 1910–13, Boston acquired its largest and most imposing municipal bath, the North Bennet Street Bath and Gymnasium, located in the North End, Fitzgerald's birthplace and the seat of his early power as ward boss. Although land was secured and a preliminary appropriation was made for this bath in 1902, it was not completed until 1910 due to fiscal constraints. By this time Italian immigrants had replaced the Irish inhabitants of the North End. Built in Italian Renaissance style, this bath was an adaptation of the Villa Medici in Rome and cost about $130,000.[26]

Baths and gymnasiums were only part of the numerous social reforms supported by "Honey Fitz" which would serve to improve the lives of Boston's ordinary citizens. Promising a "Bigger, Better, Busier Boston," he built the High School of Commerce for boys and the School of Practical Arts for girls, many playgrounds, the City Point Aquarium, and the Franklin Park Zoo, improved garbage disposal, and extended sewers and the subway to Cambridge, as well as sponsoring many other projects.[27]

During his first term Mayor Fitzgerald's largesse, his toleration of vice, and especially his abuse of patronage produced a public outcry and enraged Boston's structural reform progressives. Boston's net debt had increased from $39,418,000 in 1895 to $106,789,000 in 1907 or from $79.33 to $175.13 per capita, the largest per capita debt of any city in the United States. In response to progressive opinion, Mayor Fitzgerald created a Finance Commission made up of representatives from major Boston civic groups to investigate municipal affairs. Although the Finance Commission found corruption, especially in the awarding of contracts and job patronage, they did not uncover serious wrongdoing. Their revelations, however, were enough to seriously discredit Fitzgerald and to lead to the formation of a Committe of One Hundred, which succeeded in defeating him in his bid for reelection and electing a reform mayor, Republican George A. Hibbard.[28]

The progressive reformers also convinced the state legislature to amend Boston's charter in 1909 in an attempt to curb the power of the Irish bosses. The amended charter provided for nonpartisan elections with nomination by petition rather than by primary, increased the power of the mayor and raised the term of office from two to four years, eliminated the board of aldermen, reduced the city council to nine members elected at large, and created a permanent Finance Committee. This structural reform, however, did not keep Boston out of the hands of the bosses, for in the mayoral election of 1910, the first under the new charter, Fitzgerald, after a bitter campaign, was elected to the new, stronger mayoralty by a slim margin. His successor as mayor in 1914 was James Michael Curley, one of the United States' most notorious city bosses.[29]

Mayor Curley, like Fitzgerald, was a social reformer and big spender who continued to provide bathing facilities for the poor which increasingly were combined with gymnasiums, municipal buildings, children's playgrounds, and indoor swimming pools. In 1916 the Boston bath system included the following fifteen year-round baths:

> Dover Street Bath
> Cabot Street Bath
> North Bennet Street Bath
> Ward 16 Bath and Gymnasium
> Ward 7 Bath and Gymnasium
> Ward 9 Bath and Gymnasium
> East Boston Bath and Gymnasium
> L Street Bath and Beach

D Street Bath and Gymnasium
Copley School Baths
Curtis Hall Baths
Girls Latin School Baths
Ward 3 Bath and Gymnasium
Ward 15 Bath and Gymnasium
Ward 17 Bath and Gymnasium[30]

As in New York City, Boston's public baths were located in slums largely populated by immigrants (see map 2). But the ethnic composition of these neighborhoods was not homogeneous and was constantly changing. Boston's first bath, the Dover Street Bath, and the Ward 9 Bath served the Irish population in the South End, as did the baths located in South Boston, a predominantly Irish working-class community, and the baths located in Charlestown and Dorchester. The South End, however, was also home to Russian Jews, Italians, Poles, and African Americans. Russian Jewish immigrant Mary Antin noted in her autobiography, *The Promised Land,* that she lived on Dover Street across from the public bath, although she did not indicate whether she ever patronized the bath.[31]

The baths in the Roxbury section—the Cabot Street Bath and the Ward 17 Bath and Gymnasium—also served a mainly Irish population. Settlement house workers noted with satisfaction of the Irish in ward 17 that "two generations of living in America has . . . brought about an American standard of cleanliness." By 1905 African Americans had moved into Roxbury in considerable numbers but there was no public bath in ward 18, where they were concentrated. The Ward 7 Bath and Gymnasium near the Tenderloin district probably served a transient population. The North End, the site of the Bennet Street Bath, had originally been an Irish neighborhood but had become largely Italian, as has been noted, by the time the bath opened in 1910, although some Jews lived there also. The East Boston Bath and Gymnasium served a mixed group of Irish, Italians, and Jews.[32]

In 1909 the Baths Department had recommended that its name be changed to Municipal Gymnasia and Baths and that all beach bathing establishments be transferred from its jurisdiction to that of the Park Department. Probably as a result of these recommendations, as well as of the reorganization of Boston's government under the Amended Charter of 1909, in 1912 the Public Grounds, Baths and Music departments were

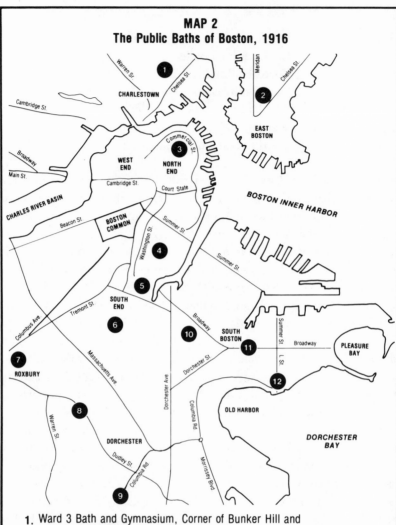

# MAP 2
## The Public Baths of Boston, 1916

1. Ward 3 Bath and Gymnasium, Corner of Bunker Hill and Lexington Streets, Charlestown
2. East Boston Bath and Gymnasium, 116 Paris Street, East Boston
3. North Bennet Street Bath and Gymnasium, North End
4. Ward 7 Bath and Gymnasium, 75 Tyler Street, central city
5. Dover Street Bath, 249 Dover Street, South End
6. Ward 9 Bath and Gymnasium, Harrison Ave. and Plympton St., South End
7. Cabot Street Bath and Gymnasium, 203 Cabot St., Roxbury
8. Ward 17 Bath and Gymnasium, Vine and Dudley Streets, Roxbury
9. Ward 16 Bath and Gymnasium, Columbia Road and Bird Street, Dorchester
10. D Street Bath and Gymnasium, South Boston
11. Ward 15 Bath and Gymnasium, Broadway between G and H Streets, South Boston
12. L Street Bath and Gymnasium, 1663 Columbia Road, South Boston

merged with the Board of Park Commissioners to form the Park and Recreation Department. The demise of the Baths Department marked the official end of the cleanliness function of Boston's municipal baths and the definite combination of baths with recreation.[33]

Unlike in New York City, there were no complaints about the lack of patronage of Boston's baths. Bath attendance rose from 581,431 in 1901 to 1,113,291 in 1915 and 1,549,480 in 1920. Part of this increase was no doubt due to the continued opening of new baths and gymnasiums, but the association of baths with recreational facilities probably best explains the growing popularity of Boston's baths, for the patronage at the Dover Street Bath, the only one without recreational facilities, steadily declined from a high of 363,755 in 1901 to 232,851 in 1915. Like New York, however, the yearly maintenance costs of Boston's bath system increased steadily, except during the administration of reform mayor Hibbard. Certainly there was some padding of the Baths Department's payroll accounts, and the Finance Commission did report some irregularities in the granting of bathhouse contracts during the first Fitzgerald administration.[34]

Boston, therefore, established a bath system that was adequate to meet existing needs and flexible enough to accommodate change. Its baths, unlike those in other cities, were not all of one type. Although it did build monumental, elaborate bathhouses, it also built several modest neighborhood gymnasiums and baths, as well as multipurpose buildings which contained baths and gymnasiums, libraries, meeting rooms, and municipal offices; its school baths were open to the general public in the evenings.

Boston's public bath movement was a reform that achieved its first success under the Brahmin Mayor Quincy, who brought to Boston many amenities which improved the lives of ordinary citizens. Quincy, in addition, for a brief time involved many disparate groups in the municipal government's efforts. Both contemporaries and modern historians considered Boston in the 1890s an especially well-governed city which had achieved many of the reforms associated with Progressivism by the time that movement was well under way. Quincy himself became a leader of the national movement for public baths. He wrote extensively on the subject in social reform periodicals and was one of the main speakers at a mass meeting on public baths held in Baltimore, Maryland, in November 1898. No doubt he was influential in convincing other American cities to follow Boston's example in providing public baths. It is ironic that Boston's progressive reformers were most concerned with efficiency, fiscal responsibility, and structural reform and left it to the city's Irish bosses, Mayors Fitzgerald and Curley, to continue the social reforms and innovations begun under Quincy, including public baths.[35]

Faced with high expenses and low patronage, Boston officially discontinued its municipal bath program in 1959. Its cleanliness baths, including those connected to recreational bathing facilities, were gradually phased out and ceased operations by the early 1970s.[36]

## The Municipal Baths of Chicago

> Women are the natural housekeepers of a great city. They have time to think, time to plan. Their intuitions are fine, and they keenly realize the necessities of the people. It is their prerogative to suggest and were this power relegated to them the work of city officials would be simplified and public funds judiciously expended.[37]

With these words the women leaders of the Free Bath and Sanitary League, the organization responsible for the successful campaign for municipal baths in Chicago, explained their actions and asserted their special abilities as women in fulfilling the role of "municipal housekeepers."

During the Progressive Era many women became involved in urban reform movements, ranging from the efforts of the settlement houses to alleviate conditions in the slums to campaigns for better schools, pure milk, and an end to the "social evil" of prostitution. Many of these women activists were, like Jane Addams (head of Hull House), members of the first generation of college-educated women, who felt an obligation to use their education for the betterment of society. Others were middle-class wives and daughters who first organized women's clubs as a means of self-education and cultural enrichment and then extended their mission to encompass improved urban services and various social reform efforts.[38]

Most of these women reformers did not consider themselves feminists and did not openly challenge women's traditional sphere of proper activity. Rather they saw their activities as a logical and natural extension of their domestic responsibilities as homemakers and mothers and saw themselves as experts in the uniquely feminine skills of housekeeping. The reforms which they advocated would produce cities that would be clean, healthful, attractive, and moral—suitable places for children and family life. As Frances Willard, the leader of the WCTU, asserted privately in 1898, "Men have made a dead failure of municipal government, just about as they would of housekeeping, and government is only housekeeping on the broadest scale." Or as Jane Addams wrote in the *Ladies Home Journal* in 1910:

If woman would keep on with her old business of caring for her house and rearing her children she will have to have some conscience in regard to public affairs lying quite outside of her immediate household. . . . They must take part in the slow up-building of that code of legislation which is sufficient to protect the home from the dangers incident to modern life.

"May we not say," she asked on another occasion, "that city housekeeping has failed partly because women, the traditional housekeepers, have not been consulted as to its multiform activities." As municipal housekeepers, women began their efforts in female-dominated institutions, such as settlement houses and women's clubs, and found that to achieve results they had to move into the male-dominated worlds of politics and economics and demand action from local and state governments. Their reform activities steadily obliterated the dichotomy between the private and public spheres.[39]

Chicago's municipal bath system, the result of the efforts of some of the city's women reformers, came closest to the bath reformers' ideal. After a brief campaign, the city opened its first modest neighborhood bathhouse in 1894 and by 1920 had constructed 21 of these small economical baths throughout the poor and working class districts. Chicago built no monumental or expensive baths, and its bath construction program was never diverted from the primary purpose of the municipal bath movement: providing easily accessible year-round bathing facilities for the poor. As the Department of Health asserted: "These baths have not been established as places of diversion and pleasure, but to promote habits of personal cleanliness by enabling those who are not provided with bathing facilities . . . to observe the fundamental rules of health and sanitation."[40]

Chicago's municipal bath movement began with the organization in 1892 of the Municipal Order League (later renamed the Free Bath and Sanitary League) by a group of Chicago women (and a few men) to improve the sanitary conditions of Chicago. To this end the league at first concentrated on such issues as the problem of streetcar spitting, street beggars and cripples, and the need for drinking fountains, park lighting, rubbish boxes, and municipal baths. Within the Municipal Order League, the chief exponent of municipal baths was Dr. Gertrude Gail Wellington, who had come to Chicago in 1892 to practice medicine. Horrified by the lack of bath facilities among Chicago's poor and anticipating public health problems as the 1893 World's Columbian Exposition approached, Dr. Wellington was converted to municipal bath advocacy. Carroll Wright's federal Bureau of Labor investigation in 1893 revealed that in Chicago's slum districts only 2.83 percent of families and 3.76 percent of individuals were living in houses or tenements with bathrooms. Wellington visited New York City, consulted with Simon Baruch, and inspected the AICP's People's Baths and then returned to Chicago to convince the Municipal Order League to mobilize its effort for the cause of municipal baths.[41]

In March 1892 the league appointed a committee of three women physicians, Wellington, Sarah Hackett Stevenson, and Julia R. Lowe, to investigate the need for public baths, assigning each to a different section of the city. Of the three, Sarah Hackett Stevenson was the most prominent. Graduating in 1874 as valedictorian from the Women's Hospital Medical College of Chicago, she was one of Chicago's leading physicians. A pioneer among women in medicine, she was the first woman member of the American Medical Association, the first woman appointed to the staff of Cook County Hospital, the first woman appointed to the Illinois State Board of Health, and the first woman instructor at Northwestern Medical College. She was also one of the founders of the Illinois Training School for Nurses. "Welcome in the upper circle of Chicago society," Stevenson was president of the Chicago Woman's Club during the World's Columbian Exposition year of 1893 and also was a member of the Twentieth Century Club and the exclusive Fortnightly Club.[42]

Julia R. Lowe was a graduate of the Chicago Homeopathic Medical College in 1881 and of the Harvey Medical College in 1895 and was therefore both a homeopathic and regular or orthodox physician. She was a dermatologist on the staff of the Mary Thompson Hospital, professor of gastroenterology at Harvey Medical College, consultant at the Women's Charity and Streeter Hospital, and attending physician at the Church Home for Aged People. The third member of the committee, Gertrude Gail Wellington, was a graduate of the New York Medical

College and Hospital, a homeopathic institution. In the 1890s homeopathy and regular medicine were converging as medical scientific knowledge advanced and the majority of homeopathic physicians moved toward an accommodation with regular practitioners. In spite of the opposition of the American Medical Association in the 1860s and 1870s, homeopathy had gained recognition and respectability; by 1903 homeopathic physicians could become members of the AMA.[43]

It is not surprising to find women physicians as leaders in the public bath movement, for those who supported the entrance of women into the profession expected that they "would become zealous advocates of public health and social morality." During the Progressive Era "their visibility in various progressive programs for health reform measured far out of proportion to their actual numbers." Their concerns ranged from industrial medicine to improving health and housing conditions in the slums and involved campaigns against tuberculosis and venereal disease.[44]

The three physicians conducted a strenuous campaign for municipal baths for Chicago. They personally approached many members of the city council, held public meetings, aroused the interest of the press, and received editorial support from the *Chicago Tribune, Herald,* and *Staats-Zeitung.* Jane Addams and the residents of Hull House added their voices to the demand for public baths, citing the fact that in 1892 in a predominantly Italian immigrant slum a third square mile adjacent to Hull House there were only three bathtubs. In a circular letter to the mayor, Hempstead Washburne, Wellington summarized the reasons that Chicago must establish a system of free public baths. Citing the success of the AICP's People's Baths of New York City, she argued that "men are vicious when dirty, as well as when hungry"; that a "free public bath will help prevent typhoid, cholera and crime"; that "the beneficent act—the giving of a free public bath—will win you the loving regard of the poor and lowly, the rich and the wise"; and that "the free public bath will inspire sweeter manners and a better observance of the law."[45]

Whether or not influenced by these arguments, which reiterated those of the bath movement, especially the linking of cleanliness to good character and to public health, Mayor Washburne endorsed the principle of municipal baths. The women also received some support from the city council, particularly from Martin Madden, chairman of the Finance Committee, who was converted to the cause of public baths. Madden later remarked:

I have been importuned both night and day for I don't know how long to lend my aid toward the construction of public bathhouses. The persuasive manner in which these ladies came upon the Council at all times and hours is what led that body to finally conclude that there was plenty of money in the treasury to be used for the purpose they desired.[46]

Martin B. Madden, an English immigrant, was a self-made businessman who had begun work in stone quarries at the age of ten and had become president of the Western Stone Company and owner of extensive real estate holdings in Chicago. A Republican, he was elected to Chicago's city council in 1889 and served there until 1897, although the reforming Municipal Voters League had tried unsuccessfully to unseat him. He was elected to Congress in 1904 and served there until his death in 1928.[47]

Before any money was appropriated for municipal baths, however, Chicago had a municipal election in which a new mayor, Carter H. Harrison, was elected. Harrison proved to be sympathetic to the cause of municipal baths, as was the press, which during February 1893 publicized the issue and urged the municipal government to build a bath for the poor. In March the council appropriated $12,000 for a bathhouse to be located on Chicago's Near West Side.[48]

The municipal government of Chicago in 1893 was similar to Boston's in that it consisted of a city council composed of seventy aldermen, two from each of the city's 35 wards, and a weak mayor elected for a two-year term. Chicago, however, had a greater amount of home rule than other major American cities. Local political machines were strong and until 1895, when the nonpartisan Municipal Voters League was organized, the city council was characterized by contemporary political scientist Delos Wilcox as "one of the most shamelessly corrupt governing bodies in the United States." "Bathhouse John" Coughlin, one of Chicago's most notoriously corrupt aldermen and ward bosses, acquired his nickname because he had been a rubber in a Turkish bath and the owner of two private bathhouses, not because of his support for the municipal bath movement. Reform efforts by the Municipal Voters League were aimed mainly at ensuring the election of honest aldermen, and the league was quite successful, although the municipal government was still plagued by graft and corruption. As Lincoln Steffens wrote in 1903, the reformers in Chicago were "half free and fighting on."[49]

Chicago's mayors were of a much higher caliber than the city council, even before reforming efforts. Hempstead Washburne, who was mayor from 1891 to 1893, had a uniformly good record and instituted such reforms as reorganization of the police department, breaking up of the gambling syndicates, and upgrading of building standards. His successor, Carter H. Harrison, was elected in 1893 to serve his fifth term as mayor of Chicago. Harrison, a very colorful and charismatic figure in Chicago politics, was born in Kentucky to a patrician southern family. A graduate of Yale University with a law degree from Transylvania University Law School, he moved in 1855 to Chicago, where he practiced law and speculated in real estate. He entered politics as a Democrat and served in Congress before he was elected mayor in 1879. Harrison was widely popular in Chicago among all ethnic groups and social classes and was recognized by all as he rode around the city on his white horse wearing his political trademark, a black felt slouch hat. Harrison had officially retired from politics at the end of his fourth term as mayor in 1887, but he emerged from his retirement in 1893 because he wanted to be mayor during the Columbian Exposition. Failing to receive the regular Democratic nomination, Harrison ran in 1893 as an independent and defeated both his Democratic and Republican opponents in spite of opposition from the political machines, the reformers, and the press. Harrison had the pleasure of presiding over the opening of the Columbian Exposition but was assassinated by a disappointed office seeker.[50]

Harrison's successors included machine politicians, reformers, and his own son, Carter Harrison II, who also served five terms. Although none of these mayors seemed actively to work for the cause of municipal baths, none of them was opposed to it either.[51]

Once the city of Chicago had appropriated the sum of $12,000 for its first municipal bath, Mayor Harrison turned planning for the bath over to Wellington and the Municipal Order League. They selected 192 Mather Street, one block north of Hull House on the Near West Side, as the site; the lot had been given to Hull House by its owner rent free for two years and Hull House offered it to the city for its first bath. Later the owner sold the land to the city. Wellington had originally projected a bath equipped with 36 showers and dressing rooms, but she was overruled by the league, which, on the advice of Stevenson and Jane Addams, head of Hull House, insisted on including a small swimming pool (20 by 30 feet) in place of more than half the showers. Apparently the swimming pool was intended to attract patrons to the bath, especially children. But the pool was not a success, probably because of its size and "the aversion of even the working people to sharing so small a body of water with each other." It was also difficult and expensive to heat the water for the pool, so in 1898 it was removed and 17 more showers were installed in its place.[52]

The Municipal Order League had recommended naming Chicago's first bathhouse after Simon Baruch, but after the assassination of Mayor Harrison the bathhouse was named in his honor instead, and a later bathhouse was named for Baruch. Chicago bathhouses were generally named in honor of prominent citizens of the city or historical figures.

The Carter H. Harrison Bath was formally opened on January 9, 1894, with Martin B. Madden as the main speaker. Other speakers included Wellington, Stevenson, and Jane Addams. The bathhouse measured 25 by 110 feet and was two stories high, with a front of Milwaukee pressed brick with brownstone trimmings. It contained a waiting room, 17 showers and dressing rooms, and 1 tub bath, was partitioned in corrugated iron, and had a small swimming pool on the first floor. The second floor contained the superintendent's living quarters. It had cost $10,856 to build, although the later removal of the swimming pool and the installation of more showers increased that cost.[53]

This first of Chicago's baths, which became a model (except for the swimming pool) for all the baths built subsequently, was much smaller, simpler, and more economical than the baths built by New York or Boston. It did not have separate facilities for men and women but instead was reserved for the exclusive use of women, girls, and small children with their mothers on two days per week. The bath patrons did not have individual control of the water and its temperature. These settings were regulated by an attendant who turned on the showers for seven to eight minutes during the twenty minutes allowed for a bath. The brief time allotted for bathing stressed the strictly functional aspect of bathing for cleanliness and allowed little time for relaxation or pleasure. The bath was free and soap and towel were also provided free of charge. Apparently neither the city government nor the Municipal Order League felt that this would pauperize its patrons.[54]

Once the Carter H. Harrison Bath was opened, the Municipal Order League, Wellington, and Madden turned their attention to Chicago's South Side, which they felt also needed a bath. They received the backing of Mayor John P. Hopkins, who requested an appropriation of $20,000, and in March 1894 the city council appropriated $12,000 for Chicago's second bath. A site 50 by 100 feet was purchased in the heart of an industrial and tenement district east of the stockyards. Wellington envisioned a much more elaborate bath for this site with separate facilities for men and women, 68 showers, a barbershop, public laundry, and soup kitchen, but these plans were altered several times.[55]

In 1895 the Municipal Order League surrendered its charter, and Chicago's bath advocates, under the leadership of Wellington, organized the Free Bath and Sanitary League to concentrate on the cause of municipal baths. Neither Stevenson nor Lowe was a trustee or an officer of this organization. The mayor of Chicago was the honorary president; Wellington was president. The vice-president was Lucy Flower, a prominent social welfare leader who with Stevenson founded the Illinois Training School for Nurses. She was also active in school reform as a member of the Chicago Board of Education, worked for the establishment of juvenile courts, and in 1894 was the first woman elected to state office in Illinois when she became a member of the Board of Trustees of the University of Illinois. Flower was an active member of the Woman's Club and had been its president in 1890–91. The working membership of the Free Bath and Sanitary League was comprised entirely of women, but there was an honorary membership of about 300 of Chicago's most prominent male citizens.[56]

It is apparent that the Chicago women involved in the municipal bath movement were an integral part of the network of women reformers in that city, which was centered in the women's clubs and settlement houses. Sarah Hackett Stevenson, Julia R. Lowe, Lucy Flower, and Jane Addams were all active members of the Chicago Woman's Club and of the more exclusive Fortnightly Club, as were several members of the Board of Trustees of the Free Bath and Sanitary League. Although Gertrude Gail Wellington does not appear to have been a member of either club, she was able to plug into this network and use its influence and support to convince the city government to inaugurate a municipal bath system.[57]

In addition to its work of advocacy of public baths, the Free Bath and Sanitary League, in the women's club tradition, also served the causes of self-improvement and sociability for its members. The league met monthly, usually at Palmer House, and enjoyed a variety of educational and other programs.[58]

With an appropriation secured for a municipal bath on the South

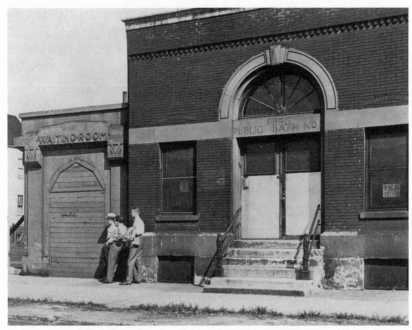

Small Public Bath, William Mavor Bath, Chicago, 1900. Source: Chicago Historical Society, ICHi–21723, photograph by Mildred Mead, 1950.

Side, the Free Bath and Sanitary League recommended that free bath facilities be provided for the North Side. However, Mary McDowell, head resident of the University of Chicago Settlement House, and the Women's Club of the settlement urged the league to propose that the next bath be located in their neighborhood, near the stockyards on the South Side. They circulated a petition throughout the Packingtown neighborhood to demonstrate to their recalcitrant alderman the people's interest in having a bath established there. These efforts were successful because Chicago's third municipal bath, the William Mavor Bath, opened there in 1900. Several subsequent baths were located on the North Side.[59]

The Free Bath and Sanitary League also recommended that the Park Commission open a summer bathing beach in Lincoln Park on the shores of Lake Michigan. The Park Commission complied with this request almost immediately and the beach opened in July 1895. In Chicago, unlike other American cities, the opening of year-round municipal baths preceded the opening of municipally supported summer bathing facilities. Wellington and the league also supported the Medical Women's

Club in its petition for the appointment of two women physicians (unnamed) to the Park Commission. In a letter to the city government Wellington noted that the older medical women had worked hard in the cause of hygiene and public health and such an appointment would be complimentary to them. She also asserted somewhat sarcastically: "I cannot imagine that either of these noble women would have boodled or flirted or smoked in the faces of the men during a board session. Their years of stability along those lines have justly placed them above princes."[60]

Chicago's second municipal bath, which was not as large as Wellington had planned, opened in April 1897 and was named in honor of Martin B. Madden. It had a waiting room, was equipped with 32 showers and dressing rooms, and had a soup kitchen in the basement. The bath was arranged so that an additional wing could be constructed which would double its capacity if the need arose. This, however, was never done. The total cost of building and equipment for this bath was $15,361.[61]

In the twenty-one years following the opening of the Martin B. Madden Bath, Chicago constructed nineteen more municipal baths in its slum districts and planned one more, which apparently was never constructed. During the construction of the Kosciuszko Bath in 1903, the people of the neighborhood "seemed bent on its destruction," and the city was compelled to station a policeman at the site during the day and two detectives there at night. The explanation for this neighborhood opposition was either that the people believed that they would be forced to bathe or that the new structure was a prison or a workhouse. At any rate when they were assured none of their assumptions was true, their opposition ceased. The construction of Chicago's other baths apparently proceeded without incident. A list of Chicago's baths is provided in table 4.1. There is no evidence that the Free Bath and Sanitary League continued to play an active role in the construction of these subsequent baths. It apparently had become the policy of the municipal government to construct an adequate bath system for the poor, and baths were opened at regular intervals until 1918 without any pressure from the bath advocates.[62]

Chicago's municipal baths, like those of New York and Boston, were located in slum neighborhoods, especially those inhabited by immigrants, or in industrial districts to serve working men (see map 3). For

Table 4.1. Municipal Baths of Chicago, 1918[a]

| | Year Opened | Cost of Land | Cost of Building and Equipment | Total Cost |
|---|---|---|---|---|
| Carter H. Harrison | 1894 | $3,750 | $16,899 | $20,649 |
| Martin B. Madden | 1897 | 5,000 | 15,361 | 20,361 |
| Twenty-second St.[b] | 1898 | — | 1,500 | 1,500 |
| Fourteenth St.[b] | 1900 | — | 3,200 | 3,200 |
| William Mavor | 1900 | 2,000 | 5,327 | 7,327 |
| Robert A. Waller | 1901 | 3,270 | 10,107 | 13,377 |
| Kosciuszko | 1904 | 3,350 | 14,410 | 17,760 |
| John Wentworth | 1905 | 2,850 | 16,703 | 19,553 |
| William B. Ogden | 1906 | 1,650 | 16,241 | 17,891 |
| Joseph M. Medill | 1906 | 1,839 | 15,419 | 17,258 |
| Theodore T. Gurney | 1906 | 5,000 | 16,730 | 21,730 |
| Thomas Gahan | 1907 | 2,189 | 17,286 | 19,475 |
| Pilsen | 1908 | 5,000 | 19,155 | 24,155 |
| Fernand Henrotin | 1908 | 5,000 | 20,043 | 25,043 |
| William Loeffler | 1909 | 3,500 | 17,561 | 21,061 |
| Simon Baruch | 1910 | 1,600 | 24,677 | 26,277 |
| Graeme Stewart | 1914 | 1,720 | 38,398 | 40,118 |
| DeWitt C. Cregier | 1915 | 3,750 | 14,794 | 18,544 |
| Kedzie Avenue | 1918 | 5,750 | 70,222[c] | 75,972 |
| Lincoln Street | 1918 | 2,500 | 42,348 | 44,848 |
| Lawler | 1918 | 16,750 | 41,375 | 58,125 |
| South Chicago[d] | in progress | 5,500 | — | 5,500 |
| Totals | | $81,968 | $437,756 | $519,724 |

[a]Chicago, Department of Health, *Report and Handbook, 1911–1918*, 1072–74; Hanger, 1317.

[b]These were shower baths for men only located in pumping stations.

[c]This bath also housed an infant welfare station, and its waiting room was large enough to serve as an auditorium.

[d]This bath was apparently never constructed.

example, the Harrison Bath, near Hull House, served the residents of a district that was largely Italian but also was home to eighteen other nationalities as well, including Russian Jews, Bohemians, and Irish. The Pilsen Bath, located in the neighborhood called Pilsen, accommodated mainly Bohemians, while the Loeffler Bath was located in the Jewish ghetto. The Cregier Bath served the Italians of Little Sicily, and the

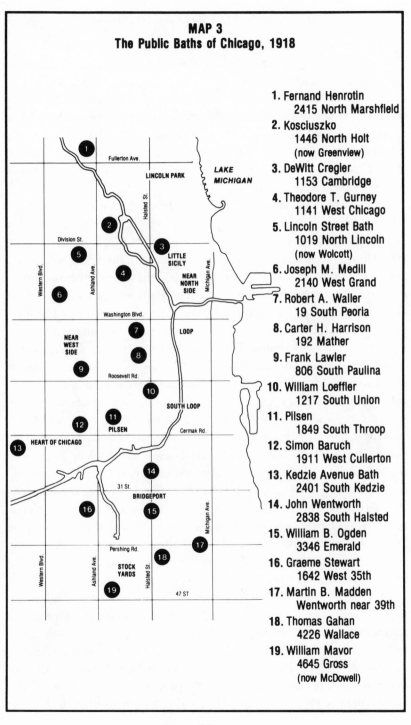

# MAP 3
## The Public Baths of Chicago, 1918

1. Fernand Henrotin
   2415 North Marshfield
2. Koscluszko
   1446 North Holt
   (now Greenview)
3. DeWitt Cregier
   1153 Cambridge
4. Theodore T. Gurney
   1141 West Chicago
5. Lincoln Street Bath
   1019 North Lincoln
   (now Wolcott)
6. Joseph M. Medill
   2140 West Grand
7. Robert A. Waller
   19 South Peoria
8. Carter H. Harrison
   192 Mather
9. Frank Lawler
   806 South Paulina
10. William Loeffler
    1217 South Union
11. Pilsen
    1849 South Throop
12. Simon Baruch
    1911 West Cullerton
13. Kedzie Avenue Bath
    2401 South Kedzie
14. John Wentworth
    2838 South Halsted
15. William B. Ogden
    3346 Emerald
16. Graeme Stewart
    1642 West 35th
17. Martin B. Madden
    Wentworth near 39th
18. Thomas Gahan
    4226 Wallace
19. William Mavor
    4645 Gross
    (now McDowell)

Lincoln Street and the Kosciuszko Bath's patrons were mainly Polish and Ukrainian immigrants. Lithuanians, Poles, Croatians, and Slovaks were the main inhabitants of the Packingtown neighborhood, the inspiration for Upton Sinclair's *The Jungle* and the site of the Mavor Bath. Irish were the majority patrons of the Medill Bath located in Bridgeport, the home of the late mayor, Richard J. Daley. Chicago's other baths were established in similar ethnic neighborhoods. Exceptions were the Gurney Bath, which was located in an industrial area, and the Waller Bath, which served the Skid Row population.[63]

During the peak use of Chicago's public baths (1894–1920) the African-American population of the city was small, although it grew rapidly from 1.3 percent in 1890 to 4.1 percent in 1920. There was an increasing concentration of African Americans on the South Side in this period but there were also important enclaves in several other sections of the city. On the South Side the Madden Bath was at the edge of the rapidly developing "black belt" and may have been patronized by African Americans, but contemporary evidence is silent on this point.[64]

The Bureau of Hospitals, Baths and Lodging Houses within the Department of Health operated Chicago's bath system, thus emphasizing the cleanliness function of these baths and their separation from any association with recreation. As we have seen, Chicago's baths were strictly utilitarian and only one, the first, had a swimming pool, which was subsequently removed. One bath, the Lincoln Street Bath, which opened in 1918, had a public laundry where the housewives of the neighborhood could do their wash. The municipal government of Chicago did maintain free swimming pools and bathing beaches, but these were controlled by the Bureau of Parks and were in no way connected to the municipal baths. The Department of Health, noting in 1910 that police were no longer stationed in bathhouses, stated: "More and more people are beginning to realize that the bath house is not a place for diversion, but for utilitarian purposes only."[65]

In spite of the functional emphasis of the Chicago baths, bath attendance, as in other cities, fluctuated greatly between the summer and winter months. For example, in 1910 bath attendance was heaviest in July with 173,222 baths taken and lightest in February with 45,517 baths. Many of Chicago's bath patrons, like those in New York City, did not have the habit of bathing regularly except in the summer months. The Department of Health attempted to educate bath patrons in the habit of bathing regularly summer and winter and observed hopefully in 1910 that "where the bathhouses have been established the longest there is the least fluctuation in the number of baths given."[66]

Chicago not only had the problem of underutilization of its baths in the winter but also that of declining overall attendance. Peak bath attendance was reached in 1910, when a total of 1,070,565 baths were taken in the 15 bathhouses in operation in that year. By 1918, with 21 bathhouses in operation, attendance had declined to 709,452. The Department of Health attributed the declining attendance in the summer months to the opening of swimming pools and free bathing beaches along the lake shore by the Bureau of Parks. Chicago's Tenement Law of 1902, which required all new tenement apartments of more than two rooms to have a private toilet, also had its effect as most builders also included a bathtub. By 1921 attendance had declined further to 524,912, and Chicago consolidated the operation of its municipal bath system within the Department of Health under the Bureau of Hospitals, Baths and Social Hygiene, which was also responsible for the operation of comfort stations, bathing beaches, and swimming pools. Thus ultimately Chicago did combine the administration of its cleanliness and recreational baths.[67]

Like New York and Boston, Chicago either converted its public baths into swimming pools or gradually closed them down after World War II. By the 1970s only one of its municipal baths remained open to serve Chicago's Skid Row residents and that too closed in 1979.[68]

Boston and Chicago each achieved a municipal bath system, but with different advocates and with different outcomes. In Boston it was a reform mayor, Josiah Quincy, who led the movement, and in Chicago it was a woman physician, Gertrude Gail Wellington, who was the primary advocate. In both cases the settlement houses lent their support to the movement. In both cities the municipal government responded to the reformers and proceeded to construct adequate bath systems. However, in Boston the baths were closely connected with recreation whereas in Chicago the baths were solely for cleanliness.

Not all cities, however, had municipal governments as willing to provide baths as New York, Boston, and Chicago. Where municipal governments were reluctant to provide this service, bath reformers turned to private philanthropy.

# 5

# Philanthropy and Progressivism: The Public Baths of Philadelphia and Baltimore

## The Public Baths of Philadelphia

> That a large city like Philadelphia should make such a poor show-
> ing in the number of free public baths may perhaps be explained by
> the fact that it is more than any other city, a "City of Homes" with
> comparatively few tenement houses and with a bath tub in nearly
> every home.
>
> —WILLIAM PAUL GERHARD

In 1900 Philadelphia was the third largest city in the United States. Its population of 1,293,697 was exceeded only by that of New York City and Chicago. Despite its size, Philadelphia never established a municipal year-round bath system, and it was only through the philanthropic efforts of a group of wealthy and prominent citizens that some public baths were constructed.[1]

This sin of omission on the part of the municipal government was usually attributed, as in the above quotation from Gerhard's *Progress of the Municipal Bath Movement in the United States,* to the fact that Philadelphia was a "city of homes" and that therefore it had little need for public baths. This rationale, however, was only partly sustained by facts. The Bureau of Labor investigation in 1893 of Philadelphia's most congested slum districts discovered that only 16.9 percent of families and 18.05 percent of individuals lived in houses or tenements with bathrooms. Although this was a much greater percentage than the approximately 3 percent with bathrooms in New York City's and Chicago's slums, it still

96

indicated a need for public baths. Further evidence of this need was supplied by the treasurer of Philadelphia's Public Baths Association, who estimated in 1899 that in the city's slum districts not one in twenty families had access to a bath. And in 1902, by actual count, the Public Baths Association found that in a typical slum block adjoining its Gaskill Street Bath there was "but one bathtub for each 155 people." Thus although the poor of Philadelphia were not as deprived of bath facilities as those in other great cities, there was certainly not a bathtub in almost every home as some reformers assumed.[2]

Although there is no doubt that Philadelphia's slums lacked bathing facilities, the fact that the city had a smaller immigrant population than New York City, Boston, and Chicago may also explain its failure to act. In 1900 about 23 percent of Philadelphia's population was foreign born, as compared to about 35 percent in the other three cities. As has been noted, almost all public baths were located in immigrant neighborhoods.[3]

The political situation in Philadelphia from 1890 to 1915 also played a role in the failure of the municipal government to build year-round baths. Lincoln Steffens in 1903 called Philadelphia "corrupt and contented" and asserted that "other American cities, no matter how bad their own condition may be, all point with scorn to Philadelphia as worse—'the worst governed city in the country.'" Delos Wilcox agreed, maintaining that it had "the reputation of being more inseparably wedded to the idols of corruption than any other great American city." Whether or not the worst, the government of Philadelphia was most certainly mired in corruption, graft, inefficiency, and fraudulent elections under its Republican political machine and bosses. One of the problems of potential progressive reformers, though, was that most of them were Republicans and strong supporters of Republican policy on the national level, especially the high tariff. They were usually unwilling to unite with Democratic reformers and had to form independent reform parties, thus splitting the reform vote. Most of the time the Republican machine and Philadelphia's "best men" coexisted comfortably.[4]

In spite of its reputation, however, Philadelphia had gone through several periods of reform during this time. In the 1870s the Committee of One Hundred had broken the notorious Gas Ring and achieved a model city charter in 1885, but the machine had returned to power in the late 1880s. In 1904–05 the Committee of Seventy succeeded in electing a reform mayor who, however, soon returned to the regular Republican organization. Again in 1911 the reformers elected a reform mayor, but many of the reforms he instituted (such as a new housing code) were opposed by the city council, which refused to appropriate the funds needed for enforcement. By the end of his term most of Philadelphia's progressive reformers had returned to the Republican party ranks.[5]

Philadelphia's progressive reformers, in their brief periods of success, were concerned mostly with structural and political rather than social reforms. The Republican machine, as Delos Wilcox noted, was in many ways "extremely negligent of the poor and unfortunate." And Philadelphia clung to its tradition of dependence on private religious and charitable organizations to solve social problems, and of resistance to the expansion of government's social welfare responsibilities.[6]

Although Philadelphia's municipal government, whether controlled by bosses or reformers, provided no municipal year-round baths, it did make ample provision for summer bathing, which was very popular among all classes of citizens. In 1885 the city had opened the first floating river bath and others followed, but they proved to be too polluted; so instead the city began to build outdoor swimming pools. By 1899 Philadelphia had 8 such swimming pools, approximately 40 by 60 feet in size, open during the summer months five days per week for men and boys and two days per week for women and girls. By 1912, the number of swimming pools had increased to 23 and the city had spent nearly $1 million in their construction.[7]

More than likely, the machine-controlled municipal government of Philadelphia built these swimming pools because of their popularity with the people but refused to build year-round baths because of the lack of popular demand for them. Reformers, with their interest in efficiency and economy, also showed no interest in year-round baths. But, if the city would not build these baths, public-spirited citizens would do so, for as Delos Wilcox cynically noted, "Philadelphia cares more for its reputation for philanthropy and Christian charity than it does for a good name for civic justice and political honesty."[8]

The public bath movement in Philadelphia began in the early 1890s almost by chance and, as in Chicago, was initiated by a woman. Sarah Dickson Lowrie, an upper class young woman who conducted a sewing class for girls in the mission building in one of Philadelphia's worst slums, was informed by her students that there was no way for them to take a bath in winter. She promptly became a public bath advocate and at a dinner party succeeded in interesting Barclay H. Warburton, editor and publisher of the Philadelphia *Daily Evening Telegraph,* in the cause of public baths. He assigned a reporter to investigate the bath situation in Philadelphia's slums in early 1895. His newspaper ran a feature article on the lack of bathing facilities in the poorer sections of Philadelphia, and Warburton proposed the raising of $50,000 for the building and equipping of public baths and washhouses for Philadelphia. He urged that a responsible group of Philadelphia citizens organize themselves to inaugurate and carry out this enterprise.[9]

The response to Warburton's proposal was the formation of the Public Baths Association of Philadelphia, which was incorporated on March 18, 1895. The purpose of the association as stated in its charter was to establish and maintain "public baths and [afford] to the poor facilities for bathing and the promotion of health and cleanliness." The association planned "to erect one or more Bath Houses and Laundries, where for a small fee persons of both sexes can obtain hot or cold baths every day of the year, and where women can do their family washing." The charter of the association did not express the hope that the bath or baths they proposed to build would serve as a model which would encourage the municipal government to build year-round baths. A few years later the treasurer of the association, however, did state in a journal article that the building of a bath through private effort would provide "a practical object-lesson" which would "do more than an attempt by mere argument to force the city councils to accept their [the bath advocates'] ideas."[10]

The Public Baths Association of Philadelphia was managed by a twelve-member board of trustees who were elected by the membership of the association for a one-year term at the annual meeting. The officers were chosen from among the trustees, who met monthly and appointed a superintendent who was responsible for the day-to-day operation of the baths. Membership in the association was restricted to any person of good character who was endorsed in writing by two members in good standing and was elected by a two-thirds vote of the members present at the annual meeting.[11]

The charter subscribers and members of the Public Baths Association, the majority of whom were on the first board of trustees, were for the most part socially prominent, wealthy, upper class Philadelphians. A few examples of the membership will illustrate this point.

The president of the first board of trustees was Eugene Delano, who

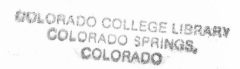

was born in Utica, New York, in 1844 and had received B.A. and A.M. degrees from Williams College. Delano had started his career as a merchant but had joined the investment banking firm Brown Brothers and Company in 1880 and was made resident partner in Philadelphia in 1894. In 1895, still with Brown Brothers, he moved to New York City, where he resided until his death in 1920. Delano was active in numerous charitable endeavors in addition to the Public Baths Association, including trusteeships of the New York Association for Improving the Condition of the Poor, the Presbyterian Hospital, the New York City Mission, and the New York Institution for the Deaf and Dumb. Although Delano moved to New York City in 1895, the year of the founding of the Public Baths Association, he continued as president of the board of trustees until 1902. As a New York City resident, Delano also served the cause of public baths as a chairman of the Public Bath Committee of the AICP.[12]

The chairman of the Finance Committee of the board of trustees and later vice-president was Barclay H. Warburton, the editor and publisher of the *Daily Evening Telegraph,* who had originated the public baths campaign in his newspaper. Born in 1866 in Philadelphia, Warburton was educated at the University of Pennsylvania and Oxford University. In 1884, when his father died, he assumed control of the newspaper that his father had founded. Warburton was married to Mary Brown Wanamaker, the daughter of John Wanamaker, the department store founder.[13]

The treasurer of the board of trustees and later chairman of the Finance Committee was Franklin B. Kirkbride. Born in Philadelphia in 1867, he was a graduate of Haverford College and son of a leading psychiatrist. Kirkbride was assistant secretary and then treasurer of the Pennsylvania Company for Insurances on Lives and Granting Annuities in Philadelphia. In 1905 he moved to New York City, where he established the Franklin B. Kirkbride Management Corporation. Kirkbride, like Delano, was active in many charitable endeavors. He played an important role in the establishment of Letchworth Village, the New York state school for the feeble-minded, and was a trustee of the Milbank Memorial Fund and the AICP (and, like Delano, a member of its Public Bath Committee). In the late 1890s and early 1900s Kirkbride wrote several journal articles on Philadelphia's public baths and lectured frequently on the subject.[14]

Delano's successor as president of the board of trustees was Edward B. Smith, a prominent Philadelphia banker and financier who was head of his own investment banking firm. Born in Philadelphia in 1861, he was a graduate of the University of Pennsylvania. Smith too was involved in many charitable enterprises, most notably the Pennsylvania Society to Protect Children from Cruelty and the Tuberculosis Camp, and was a director of the City Trusts, which managed the Girard Estates.[15]

Kirkbride's successor as treasurer of the board of trustees was his nephew Arthur V. Morton. Morton was born in Philadelphia in 1874 and was a graduate of the University of Pennsylvania. Morton was employed by the Pennsylvania Company for Banking and Trusts and eventually became its president in 1924. His charitable activities include trusteeship of the Pennsylvania Hospital.[16]

Sarah Dickson Lowrie was also a member of the original board of trustees. "One of Old Philadelphia's more famous spinsters," she was born in 1870 and attended the Farmington School in Connecticut. Throughout her long life (she died in 1957) she was involved in many varied activities. She was a founder of the Philadelphia Junior League and the Lighthouse Settlement. She was a columnist for the *Philadelphia Evening Ledger* and on the staff of the *Ladies Home Journal.* A leader in the Philadelphia movement for women's suffrage, she led the first women's suffrage parade in that city. She was also interested in historic preservation and headed the restoration of Pennsbury, William Penn's country home, and wrote a book on the history of Strawberry Mansion, a Philadelphia home from the colonial period. When she resigned from the board of trustees of the Public Baths Association in 1908, the trustees noted in their minutes that it was "owing greatly to Miss Lowrie's untiring efforts that the money was raised to build the first bathhouse."[17]

Probably the best-known member of the board of trustees of the Public Baths Association and the wealthiest (he was on the *New York Tribune*'s list of American millionaires in 1901) was Charlemagne Tower. Tower, whose money was inherited from his father of the same name, was a diplomat, author, and lawyer-businessman. Born in Philadelphia in 1849, he was a graduate of Harvard University. After a career in business and law, he served as ambassador to Austria, Russia, and Germany between 1897 and 1908. In all these posts he lived and entertained on a very lavish scale. Tower's avocation was history, and he was president of the Historical Society of Pennsylvania and the author of a number of historical essays and one book, *The Marquis de Lafayette in the American Revolution.*[18]

Other members of the board of trustees were equally prominent and were members of Philadelphia's leading families. Names such as Drexel, Wanamaker, Weightman, Paul, and Harrison appear as either trustees or donors. It is obvious that Philadelphia's public bath advocates were patrician reformers who were active in a variety of charitable enterprises, as well as the Public Baths Association. Until 1910 the board of trustees also usually, but not always, included, in addition to Sarah Lowrie, three or four women who cannot be further identified. From that year forward all the trustees were men. One or two physicians and a minister were also frequently members. Generally the trustees contributed generously to the association with yearly gifts ranging up to $1,000. Money was also raised by staging benefits, such as a theatrical event at the New Century Drawing Rooms in 1902 which netted $300.[19]

With the incorporation of the Public Baths Association and fund raising under way, plans proceeded for the construction of the first bath. A site on Gaskill Street in Southwark, one of the oldest and most thickly populated sections of the city and "one of the vilest Jewish immigrant neighborhoods," was purchased for $5,750. Plans for the bath itself were strongly influenced by the AICP's People's Baths in New York City because some of the trustees inspected those baths as well as a bathhouse in Yonkers, New York, built in compliance with New York's mandatory bath law. As a result they decided that no swimming pool would be included. Originally a large bath with 57 showers was planned at a total cost of about $29,000. However, such a large bath could not be built for that price so ultimately the association had to settle for a smaller one. They did decide to include a public laundry in the bath, which was an innovation, for whereas many European baths had laundries, none in the United States did at this time.[20]

The Gaskill Street Bath was formally opened on April 20, 1898, with several hundred of Philadelphia's "best and most distinguished citizens" present. The two-and-one-half-story bath contained 26 showers and 1 bathtub for men, 14 showers and 3 bathtubs for women, a public laundry in the basement, and living quarters for the superintendent on the second floor. Located on a 40 by 60-foot lot, it was in colonial style of red brick trimmed with dark mortar. The total cost of lot, bathhouse, and equipment was $29,903, quite close to the original budget.[21]

There was no question in the minds of the trustees of the Public Baths Association that a fee should be charged for the use of the bath. A five

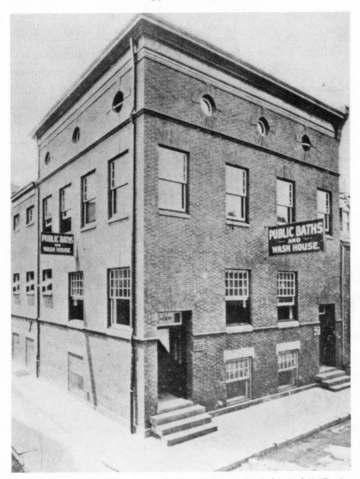

Gaskill Street Public Baths and Wash House. Built by Public Baths
Association of Philadelphia, 1898. Source: G. W. W. Hanger, "Pub-
lic Baths in the United States," U.S. Department of Commerce and
Labor, *Bulletin of the Bureau of Labor* 9 (1904), plate no. 160. Econom-
ics and Public Affairs Division, New York Public Library, Astor,
Lenox, and Tilden foundations.

cent fee was charged for a shower bath, ten cents for a tub bath, both with
towel and soap; children under ten with their parents were admitted free.
The fee for use of the laundry was five cents per hour. The association
pointed out that it cost five cents for a glass of beer and declared that "the
poor man liked to be clean even to the extent of denying himself a glass of

beer in exchange for a bath." It also stated that the small charge prevented "the humiliation that arises in the self-respecting poor when receiving alms" and would not "'pauperize' its beneficiaries" as "each one pays for what he gets." The association expressed the hope that the fees would eventually make the bathhouse self-supporting and this hope did become a reality in 1910. The bath was open every day of the year, including Sundays and holidays.[22]

The Public Baths Association deemed the Gaskill Street Bath an immediate success, noting expansively that it was "patronized by all nationalities, Hebrews, Italians, Germans, Irish, English, Japanese, Hungarians, as well as Americans, black and white." The majority of patrons, however, were Jewish. The total number of bathers in 1898 was 21,656, or an average of 88 per day, although the capacity of the bath was over 900 per day; only 256 persons patronized the laundry. As in other cities, the patronage also varied greatly between winter and summer; in July 1898 there were 4,945 bathers and in November the total was 787.[23]

The Public Baths Association, although pleased with the modest success of the bath, took steps to increase patronage. In 1899, it had posters printed advertising the bath and requested that neighborhood stores, barbershops, saloons, and charitable organizations display them. Thousands of cards were distributed from house to house and in the streets. In addition, "an advertising wagon with descriptive signs and a large bell attached was kept on the streets thirty days during the early summer." These efforts apparently were effective, for in 1902 the number of bathers at the Gaskill Street Bath had increased to 62,377, or an average of 170 per day, and laundry patrons totaled 1,156.[24]

The association was very proud of its public laundry equipped with hot and cold water, washtubs, drying closets, ironing boards, and irons. Its treasurer, Franklin B. Kirkbride, remarked that the laundry's patrons ranged "from the men who come on Sundays to wash their only set of under-clothing, to the small shopkeepers who send their servants to do the family washing and ironing." The association also was gratified to report that the Gaskill Street Bath had "visitors from St. Louis, Chicago, New York, Baltimore, and other leading cities, with the result of stimulating the bath-house movement throughout the country."[25]

In 1900 the Public Baths Association noted that the Gaskill Street Bath was becoming more self-supporting, with fees covering 64 percent of the expenses. Because of this they felt that "with a clear conscience funds

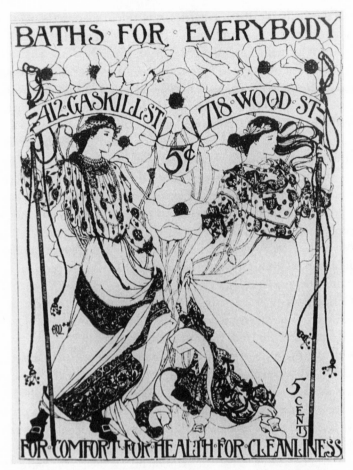

Advertising Poster by Ellen Macauley for Philadelphia's Public Baths.
Source: W. L. Ross, "Cleanliness and Its Advertisement," *Charities* 12
(Apr. 2, 1904), 334.

may be asked for the building of Public Bath No. 2," and a fund-raising
campaign was begun. In urging support of a second bath the association
observed that "the bath house movement throughout the country" was
growing rapidly and expressed the hope that "Philadelphia will not only
keep abreast, but lead in this very important branch of moral and material progress.[26]

Fund raising and plans for the second bathhouse proceeded, and land
was purchased at 718 Wood Street for $2,328 in 1901. The neighborhood

around this bath, Northern Liberties, was a slum that was home to Russian and Austro-Hungarian Jews and Irish immigrants. The Wood Street Bath, which formally opened on March 30, 1903, was somewhat smaller than the first bath, having 24 showers for men and 6 for women as well as a public laundry. It too was built in colonial style and cost approximately $20,000. The opening reception and tea for contributors and members of the Public Baths Association was, like the first one, a lively social affair and caused quite a stir in the neighborhood as the *Philadelphia Press* reported: "Broughams, with liveried coachmen and footmen on the boxes, arrived in the rain through streets they never traveled before and deposited women prominent in social circles at the quaint little colonial building. The inhabitants looked in amazement from front windows at the procession."[27]

Also in 1903 the Public Baths Association built a separate laundry and small bath exclusively for women opposite the Gaskill Street Bath, which thereafter was reserved for men. The reason was that women patrons of the Gaskill bath objected to the increasing use of the bath and especially of the laundry by vagrant men. This one-story bath was also of colonial design and cost, with land, $8,998 to build and equip.[28]

With the opening of these two new baths in 1903 the association continued its widespread advertising of the public baths. Calendars, posters, cards, and free tickets were liberally distributed to individuals in the street, to private houses, places of business, and charitable organizations. The local press, especially Barclay Warburton's *Daily Evening Telegraph,* also cooperated with the baths association by printing numerous feature articles as well as free advertisements for the public baths.[29]

This policy of advertising achieved results, for in 1907 bath patronage had increased to 149,160, or an average of 408 baths per day, in the three baths in operation, although this patronage did not begin to tax the baths' capacity. Laundry patronage also increased to 4,993. By this year also, the three baths were almost self-supporting: 92 percent of the operating expenses of $10,416 were met by the fees charged. Encouraged by decreasing costs and continuing increases in patronage, the Public Baths Association of Philadelphia built another bath for the poor, which opened on November 12, 1912. This bath, located at 1203 and 1205 Germantown Road, was larger than Philadelphia's other public baths, with 62 showers for men and 8 for women. It was "in the heart of a poor district" in Kensington, a working class industrial area predominantly inhabited by

Irish and English immigrants but also home to many other ethnic groups. Nearly 400 persons contributed to the building fund for this bath in amounts ranging from $1 to the $2,500 donated by two officers of the association, Edward B. Smith, president and George L. Harrison, Jr., vice-president.[30]

As the fees charged for the baths made them self-supporting and contributions to the association continued, in 1915 the trustees were able to enlarge the Wood Street Bath to contain 70 showers.[31]

Whereas bath reformers in other cities felt that their work was completed by 1920 and built almost no more baths after that date, the Public Baths Association of Philadelphia built two more public baths during the 1920s. Why they did this is not entirely clear, although they continued to believe that public baths were needed. A most important reason, however, was their financial success. In 1915 they received a $5,000 bequest from Elizabeth Shippen. By that year the existing baths were not only self-supporting but also had begun to show a profit of $281. By 1921 the surplus of revenues after expenses had increased to $20,818. Contributions had also grown steadily, reaching a peak of $10,332 in 1916 and averaging $6,000 to $7,000 per year in the 1920s.[32]

In 1921 the Public Baths Association opened a large public bath at Passyunk Avenue and Wharton Street, containing 96 showers, at a cost of $74,344. This bath was located in South Philadelphia in a neighborhood inhabited mainly by Italian immigrants. Even after building this bathhouse, the association recorded in 1922 that it held investments totaling $59,000 in value. In 1924 it therefore decided to build another bathhouse in Kensington, a major manufacturing area where its Germantown Avenue Bath was well patronized. This bath, located at 1808–14 Hazzard Street, opened in 1928 and was the largest and most expensive bath built by the association. It contained 107 showers and cost $108,798.[33]

Although Philadelphia had a sizable African-American population— 62,613 people, who made up almost 5 percent of the total population in 1900, and 134,229, or 7.4 percent, in 1920—the Public Baths Association constructed no baths in African-American neighborhoods. But the Gaskill Street Baths were on the border of a major African-American district. Like bath reformers in other cities, the association focused its efforts on immigrant neighborhoods (see map 4).[34]

As these new baths opened, patronage reached a peak of 530,964 in 1928, as did the surplus of revenues over expenses of $15,339. Never-

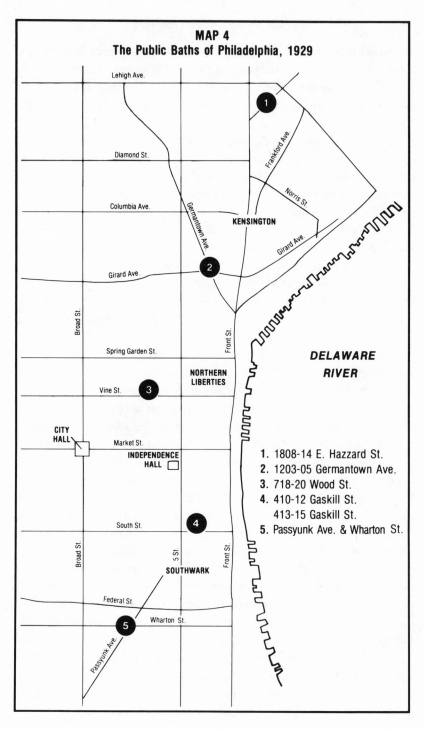

# MAP 4
## The Public Baths of Philadelphia, 1929

Lehigh Ave.

Diamond St.

Frankford Ave.

Norris St.

Columbia Ave.

Germantown Ave.

**KENSINGTON**

Girard Ave.

Girard Ave.

Broad St.

Front St.

Spring Garden St.

**DELAWARE RIVER**

**NORTHERN LIBERTIES**

Vine St.

**CITY HALL**

Market St.

**INDEPENDENCE HALL** ▢

1. 1808-14 E. Hazzard St.
2. 1203-05 Germantown Ave.
3. 718-20 Wood St.
4. 410-12 Gaskill St.
   413-15 Gaskill St.
5. Passyunk Ave. & Wharton St.

South St.

Broad St.

5 St.

Front St.

**SOUTHWARK**

Federal St.

Wharton St.

Passyunk Ave.

theless, beginning in 1929, both patronage and surpluses began to decline and by 1932 the surplus had become a deficit of $10,667. The trustees attributed declining patronage to the widespread unemployment caused by the Great Depression and did their share to help in 1930 by hiring unemployed men in the bathhouses to paint and do small repairs and in 1931 by contributing $1,000 to the Committee for Unemployment Relief. Throughout the 1930s patronage declined, deficits mounted, and contributions diminished, although the association urged contributors to increase their donations.[35]

In 1942 the trustees considered the question of whether the Public Baths Association should be liquidated but decided to carry on for a while longer, although in that year they closed the Gaskill Street Baths. In their fund-raising efforts they cited the 1940 census, which revealed that 14.3 percent of dwellings in Philadelphia still lacked private bathing facilities, but to no avail. Yearly contributions dwindled to a few hundred dollars. In 1943 they closed the Hazzard Street Bath, "which [had] shown continuing deficits in each year since it opened in 1928." In 1944 and 1945 the trustees sold the bathhouses which had closed, and in 1946 they voted to cease operations, stating that there was no longer a need for "this charitable enterprise." They closed the two remaining bathhouses in 1948 and sold them to the city of Philadelphia. After arranging for pensions for bathhouse employees and donating their assets of $69,632 to the Philadelphia Foundation, the Public Baths Association of Philadelphia ceased to exist on January 11, 1950.[36]

Although the city of Philadelphia built no public baths for its poorer citizens, the city's patrician bath reformers cannot be faulted for lack of sustained devotion to the cause. From its inception in 1895 the Public Baths Association raised large sums of money, built public baths, and continued to build them after the movement had lost vigor in other cities. Philadelphia's bath reformers were also active in the national movement; the superintendent of the baths or a member of the association usually served on the board of directors of the national organization, the American Association for Promoting Hygiene and Public Baths. Some trustees' interest in the cause of public baths spanned generations and lasted a lifetime. The last president of the board of trustees was Edward B. Smith, Jr., who served from 1929 to 1950. His father had been president from 1902 to 1918. Arthur V. Morton was treasurer from 1905 until his death in

1949, and Barclay H. Warburton, one of the founders of the association in 1895, voted with the other trustees to dissolve it in 1950.[37]

## The Public Baths of Baltimore

> Our economy of management of baths and laundries, our freedom from political or personal influence in making appointments of employees, our careful sanitary regulations as to cleanliness, and withal the large success resulting, have given our city a national reputation in this department.[38]
>
> —FREE PUBLIC BATH COMMISSION OF BALTIMORE

Although Baltimore was somewhat later than other American cities in establishing its small municipal bath system, once the system was founded it compensated for its late start by the efficiency of its operation and the continuing and unflagging interest of its bath advocates. The leaders of the Baltimore public bath movement not only strongly urged the city to build municipal baths in the early 1890s but served as charter members of the Free Public Bath Commission, supervising Baltimore's baths while they were being constructed and after the system was completed.

In Baltimore the public bath system was not a clear-cut result of urban progressive reform or of simple private philanthropy. Although reformers controlled the municipal government between 1895 and 1910, they were not responsive to the demands for municipal baths by the leading bath proponents, some of whom were themselves progressive leaders. Instead, Baltimore acquired a public bath system largely through the generosity of its wealthiest citizen, Henry Walters, who donated four public bathing facilities to the city, which then agreed to operate them.[39]

The public bath movement began in Baltimore in 1893, when the Reverend Thomas M. Beadenkopf, pastor of the Canton Congregational Church, located in a poorer section of East Baltimore, saw the need for a summer bathing beach in the area. He solicited funds from his wealthier parishioners and other interested citizens and opened a "bathing shore" at Canton in July that was Baltimore's first public bathing site. The next year Beadenkopf convinced Baltimore officials that the city should take over and operate Canton Beach, and $500 was appropriated for this purpose.[40]

Also in 1894 Beadenkopf approached some of Baltimore's prominent citizens and persuaded them that there was a need for year-round baths as well as a summer bathing beach and asked them to join him in urging city officials to establish permanent baths. Mayor Ferdinand Latrobe's response was the creation of a Bath Commission to study the question and make recommendations. He also requested that Beadenkopf and the others serve as members. The Bath Commission, as it finally was constituted, included the presidents of the first and second branches of the city council; William H. Morriss, secretary of the YMCA; James Carey Thomas, a physician; Beadenkopf, who was appointed secretary; and Eugene Levering, who was president. Since ultimately the leadership of both Beadenkopf and Levering was crucial to the success of Baltimore's public bath movement, it is appropriate to review their respective backgrounds.[41]

Beadenkopf, of German descent, was born in 1855. A graduate of Johns Hopkins University in 1880 and Yale Divinity School in 1885, he became pastor of the Canton Church in Baltimore in 1891. Once the bathing beach at Canton was established, Beadenkopf became a staunch advocate of municipal baths, both summer and year-round, and devoted the rest of his life to that cause. He was a member of Baltimore's first Free Public Bath Commission and in 1902 was appointed by the commission to be superintendent of Baltimore's municipal baths, a full-time, salaried position. He served in this capacity until his death in 1915. He was also one of the founders of the American Association for Promoting Hygiene and Public Baths and was elected vice-president of the association at its first meeting in 1912.[42]

Born in Baltimore in 1845, Eugene Levering was the descendant of German immigrants who came to America in 1685. He did not attend college and instead went to work in his father's grocery and importing business. He moved from this business to banking and eventually became president and chairman of the board of the National Bank of Commerce of Baltimore. Levering was listed in the Baltimore Social Register but was most active in educational, religious, charitable, and philanthropic endeavors. He was a deacon in his Baptist church and treasurer of the Maryland Baptist Association. He also served as director of the Charity Organization Society and as president of the Baltimore Association for Improving the Condition of the Poor. He was one of the founders of the American Red Cross and a member of its board of directors and was a trustee of George Washington and Johns Hopkins universities. He donated Levering Hall to Johns Hopkins and in 1893 established Levering House for Men in Baltimore, an institution similar to the Mills Hotels for homeless men in New York City. In addition to his activity in many of the reform movements of the day, Levering was a strong proponent of public baths and was appointed president of the Free Public Bath Commission of Baltimore when it was created in 1900 to administer the Baltimore baths. He served in this post until his death in 1928 at the age of eighty-two.[43]

Baltimore's first Bath Commission, of which Levering was also the president, began its work in 1894. At its urging the city opened two other bathing beaches to the public in 1894 but took no action on the recommendation that permanent year-round baths be established. In 1895 Beadenkopf toured Europe to study the bath systems there, especially those in Germany and England, and reported to the Bath Commission on his findings. Again in 1896, 1897, and 1898 the Bath Commission urged the municipal government to construct all-season baths but to no avail.[44]

It is unclear why the city government was reluctant to build municipal baths. In 1895 the Reform League, which had been established in 1885, finally succeeded in overthrowing the Democratic machine that had controlled the city since 1867. Although there was no large-scale corruption or scandal during the reign of the Democratic boss, Isaac Freeman Rasin, the city of Baltimore was poorly governed. For example, the school system was one of the worst in the country, and Baltimore, with its population of over one-half million people, had no sewer system. The mayor was usually a member of Baltimore's upper class, which was friendly to the machine but not subservient to it. Ferdinand Latrobe, a member of an old Baltimore family, served seven terms as mayor from 1875 to 1895. The chairman of Baltimore's Reform League was Charles J. Bonaparte, a Progressive Republican and friend of Theodore Roosevelt, who later appointed him to his cabinet. The Reform League, which was a Republican-reform coalition, succeeded in gaining control of the city council in 1894 and of the mayoralty in 1895, when a Republican businessman, Alcaeus Hooper, was elected.[45]

Thus, when the Baltimore Bath Commission made its recommendations in the late 1890s, the city's municipal reformers had achieved victory over the machine. But the Baltimore reform movement in general was not as sympathetic to the cause of municipal baths as the movements led in New York City by Mayor William L. Strong and in Boston by Josiah Quincy.

One reason for the lack of response from Baltimore's progressive-reform government may be that the need for other urban services was more pressing. And in fact the need for municipal baths was not as great in Baltimore as in other cities. Next to Philadelphia, Baltimore had more residents living in single-family houses than any other major city. However, the federal Bureau of Labor investigation of slum conditions in Baltimore in 1893 had revealed that only 7.35 percent of the families and 9.21 percent of individuals in slums had bathrooms in their houses or tenements. Although these percentages were higher than for most other cities, they still indicated a real lack of bathing facilities.[46]

Another reason may have been Baltimore's comparatively small immigrant population. In 1890, its foreign-born population comprised less than 16 percent of its total population, while in New York, Boston, and Chicago the foreign born reached or exceeded 35 percent of the total population. However, in 1890 Baltimore did have the largest African-American population of any city except Washington, D.C. The preponderance of African Americans among Baltimore's slum population may also account for the city's official reluctance to build public baths; when it was later suggested that a public bath be constructed for "colored people," city officials were opposed and revealed their prejudice by maintaining that they "would not use the baths, that their maintenance would be a waste of the city's money."[47]

Joseph L. Arnold has also pointed out Baltimore's tradition of privatism, wherein residents or building contractors often paid for various urban amenities, such as public squares, police and fire call boxes, fountains, sidewalks, and even school buildings, which would then be maintained by the municipal government. Finally, there is no evidence of demand for public baths on the part of those citizens of Baltimore for whom the baths were intended, and this may also account for the municipal government's indifference.[48]

Although Baltimore's Bath Commission under the presidency of Eugene Levering was rebuffed by the municipal government, it did succeed in arousing public interest in the question of municipal baths and in securing the support of the Maryland Public Health Association.[49]

In November 1898, at a state conference on charities and correction, the Maryland Public Health Association sponsored an open meeting on public baths. The main speakers were Mayor Josiah Quincy of Boston and Franklin Kirkbride of the Public Baths Association of Philadelphia.

Each spoke on the progress of the public bath movement in his city. Eugene Levering also spoke on the necessity for year-round baths in Baltimore and urged their immediate establishment either by the municipal government, as was done in Boston, or through public donations, as was the case in Philadelphia.[50]

The response to this public meeting was disappointing, producing no reaction from the city government and few donations from the public. The Bath Commission then determined to solicit the editorial support of Baltimore's newspapers as well as to advertise in them for the cause. The following notice appeared in Baltimore's daily newspapers early in December 1898:

### PUBLIC BATHS
*Shall Baltimore Have Them?*

The recent meeting at McCoy Hall at which Mayor Quincy of Boston and F. B. Kirkbride of Philadelphia showed what is being done in those cities in the matter of Public Baths, aroused great interest. Baltimore's showing was almost grotesque in contrast.

The question is "Shall Baltimore continue to occupy this position?"

Boston spends $35,000 annually for public baths; New York, $48,000; Philadelphia, Chicago, Buffalo, Detroit, and even Wilmington spend large sums for this purpose. Baltimore appropriates $500 per year toward maintenance of summer baths. Baths open all the year round, equipped with hot and cold water, and accessible to all who are now deprived of these privileges, are a necessity. In some sections of our city, bathrooms are not provided in 90 percent of homes.

The Baltimore Commissioners are ready to open such baths if money is provided. They have secured in cash and pledges about $600 but it will take $2,000 to carry out even the most modest plan.

Subscriptions to this fund are earnestly solicited and may be sent to Eugene Levering. . . .

BY ORDER OF THE COMMISSION

At the same time, editorial support was also forthcoming. The Baltimore *Sun,* for example, endorsed the advertisement and the idea of municipal baths. It felt that if Baltimore could not raise as large a fund as New York City or Boston "through public appropriations or private subscriptions, it ought to be entirely feasible to make a beginning without further delay and to lay the foundations for a more elaborate system in the future." It hoped that "civic pride, as well as civic interest, may make prompt and generous response to the commission's appeal" and noted that "public baths may be regarded in the light of home missions for the improvement of physical and moral conditions."[51]

In spite of the advertisement and the editorial endorsements, again there was little response on the part of the citizens of Baltimore and none from the municipal government to the pleas of the Bath Commission. The Bath Commission then began to approach Baltimore's wealthier citizens individually for contributions. It found Henry Walters, the railroad magnate, very receptive and much interested. Walters, who had been contacted by Beadenkopf, asked for detailed information on public baths. The Bath Commission sent Beadenkopf to Boston, New York City, and Chicago to study the bath systems of these cities.[52]

On February 1, 1899, the Bath Commission submitted its report to Henry Walters. The commission recommended that four baths be established in Baltimore's most congested areas and listed the proposed sites in order of their importance: Southeast Baltimore, Old Town, Southwest Baltimore, and South Baltimore. It asserted that the purpose of the baths should be cleanliness only and that they therefore should be equipped with showers and tubs, but not swimming pools. At the suggestion of Dr. Edward M. Hartwell, the Boston bath reformer, they stated that the baths should be modeled on the small, simple German volksbaden and estimated that this type of bath would cost about $12,000 to build and $1,500 per year to maintain.[53]

On February 2, 1899, Walters responded to the commission's report by advising that he was "willing to erect three baths in Baltimore at a cost not exceeding $15,000 each, the baths to be known as the 'Walters Public Baths.'" When these baths were completed, they were to be turned over to the municipal government for operation and maintenance. Walters requested that the Bath Commission secure lots for the baths and prepare plans and specifications for his signature. Thus, the Baltimore bath advocates, after five years of agitation, had found a benefactor who would provide the city with the nucleus of a public bath system.[54]

Henry Walters had been born in Baltimore in 1848. A Catholic, he received a B.A. and an M.A. from Georgetown University in 1869 and 1871. After two years' study at Lawrence Scientific School at Harvard, he was awarded the B.S. degree. Already wealthy through inheritance, Walters became a railroad capitalist who through consolidation gained control of 10,000 miles of railroad. Chairman of the board of the Louisville and Nashville line, he was "said to be the richest man in the South." He was a major art collector and he went to Europe every year to buy art of all kinds. As his father had done, Walters bequeathed his collection, galleries, and one-quarter of his estate as an endowment for maintenance of his collection to the City of Baltimore, and the resulting Walters Art Gallery remains a major cultural force in the city.[55]

Walters was not involved in progressive reform either in Baltimore or on the national level and attributed his interest in public baths to a trip he had taken to Egypt, where he had become aware of the relationship of cleanliness and sanitation to public health. He said:

I was greatly impressed with the filth and squalor in the poorer sections of the towns, and it was pointed out to me that these sections were the places where the greatest epidemics started. On returning home I made some investigation, which disclosed the fact that in the poorer sections of Baltimore, especially in the neighborhoods where the foreign peoples dwelt, there was room for great improvement in sanitary conditions. When you consider that in some houses from 100 to 150 people are congregated without means for keeping clean you can realize, as I did, what a boon a public bath house would be.[56]

Once Walters had made his offer to donate three baths to the City of Baltimore, the Bath Commission acted quickly to produce the required plans and specifications. They dispatched two of their members, Beaden-kopf and William H. Morriss, to Philadelphia to study its year-round baths. Their report, coupled with statistics on the cost of baths in other cities, forced the Bath Commission to revise its estimated cost of the baths upward to $20,000–$25,000 each. The commission, therefore, went to Walters and asked him to donate two baths instead of three. Walters agreed to do so and increased his gift to $50,000 for two baths. The study of the Philadelphia baths also probably convinced the Bath Commission that public laundries should be included in public bath-houses, as they were in Philadelphia.[57]

The City of Baltimore passed ordinances agreeing to accept the lots and buildings for the baths and laundries and to maintain them. The city was to be allowed to dispose of the buildings and lots, if necessary, but must use the money obtained for the erection of public baths and laundries.[58]

Plans proceeded quickly for the construction of Walters Bath No. 1, and it was formally opened on May 18, 1900. At the opening ceremony Henry Walters presented the keys and deed to the bath to the acting

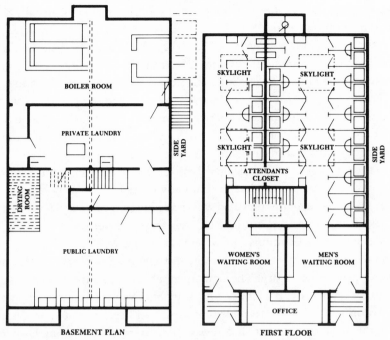

Walters Bath No. 1, Baltimore, Maryland. Floor plan, typical small bath-house. Source: G. W. W. Hanger, "Public Baths in the United States," U.S. Department of Commerce and Labor, *Bulletin of the Bureau of Labor* 9 (Washington, D.C., Government Printing Office, 1904), Plate 130.

mayor, expressing the hope that the city "will run the bath houses on the good old democratic principle of the greatest good to the greatest number." The gift was accepted with pleasure and grateful appreciation.[59]

Walters Bath No. 1 was located at 131 South High Street in an old and crowded section of the city inhabited mostly by Jewish immigrants and close to the waterfront. A "simple but elegant structure" built on a 46 by 70-foot lot, it was equipped with 18 showers for men, 5 showers and 2 tubs for women, and a public laundry in the basement. The opening of the bath was hailed editorially by the *Baltimore Sun,* which declared the bath to be complete in every way. It asserted that "the thanks of the whole city are due to the benefactor and his intelligent and experienced advisors in the matter." The bath was popular with the city's transient male population, especially with seamen and fishermen. Eventually, the Bath Commission restricted use of its laundry to men only, and the bath became a place where itinerants could bathe and wash their clothes, usually the ones they were wearing.[60]

With the opening of Walters Bath No. 1, the city established the Free Public Bath Commission of Baltimore to replace the original Bath Commission, first organized in 1894. The new commission had seven members appointed by the mayor who were to serve without pay. They were empowered to maintain and operate all public baths, which included the outdoor beach baths as well as the new indoor bath, and to make rules and regulations regarding them.[61]

Three members of the original Bath Commission were appointed to the new commission, so that the bath advocates had the opportunity to administer the facilities they had worked so long to obtain. The president of the new commission, as of the old, was Eugene Levering. Also retained from the original commission were William H. Morriss, who was appointed vice-president and treasurer, and Thomas M. Beadenkopf, who was appointed secretary. The new members included three physicians, John S. Fulton, Joseph Gichner, and Mary Sherwood. The latter, who was active in many Baltimore reform groups, had been educated at Vassar and the University of Zurich and was on the staff of the Evening Dispensary for Working Women and Girls in Baltimore, which maintained a small public bath. The seventh member was George W. Corner, Jr., a member of the city council.[62]

Rather ironically, one of the first decisions which the Free Public Bath Commission made was that the new baths should not be absolutely free. Instead, as in Philadelphia, small fees were charged for the use of the baths and the laundry—three cents for soap and towel, one cent for young children with a parent, and two and one-half cents per hour for laundry privileges. The Bath Commission felt that a small charge was more satisfactory to the bath patrons and rendered them "more self-respecting."[63]

While Walters Bath No. 2 was under construction in 1901, the Bath Commission began to urge the city to build outdoor swimming pools in its public parks. It reiterated this recommendation until 1905, when the first outdoor swimming pool was opened. The Baltimore Bath Commission, therefore, was not unconcerned with the recreational aspects of bathing but believed that they should be separated from the hygienic.[64]

Also, in 1901 the Bath Commission appointed Beadenkopf to the full-time salaried position of superintendent of the public baths and secretary of the commission. He was replaced on the commission by Morris Soper, a young Baltimore-born lawyer and judge who was active in the Reform League and various charities. A majority of the members of the Bath Commission were associated with various charitable and reform groups, although only Soper was active in the Reform League (the reform coalition that had won control of the municipal government in 1895).[65]

During 1901, patronage of the Walters Bath No. 1 was 70,000, a number which the Bath Commission believed indicated that the facilities met "a real need felt by many persons in our city." It expressed concern, however, over the disparity between summer and winter patronage, noting that usage for January 1901 had been 1,855 as opposed to 8,449 the following June, an inevitable problem to public bath advocates.[66]

In 1901 Henry Walters offered to build the city a third public bath at a cost of $25,000 upon the completion of Walters Bath No. 2. There was a delay, however, in the construction of bath no. 3. Beadenkopf recommended that this bath should be for the use of "colored people" on the assumption that the white people of Baltimore would not be willing to use a common bath with African Americans, and that "our colored Americans should have an equal chance with white people for cleanliness and recreation." But city officials felt that African Americans would not use the bath and that its maintenance would be a waste of the city's money. Beadenkopf's point of view, however, ultimately prevailed, and in 1903 land was purchased in the most crowded and unhealthy black section of Baltimore for bath no. 3. James B. Crooks has pointed out that this public bath was one of the few exceptions to the general discrimination against African Americans in the reforms instituted in Baltimore during the Progressive Era.[67]

In the meantime, Walters Bath No. 2, located in a manufacturing neighborhood, was opened in April 1902. Built in "free colonial style," it had 20 showers for men, 6 showers and 2 tubs for women, and a public laundry for the use of women only. Its patrons were mostly Lithuanian immigrants. In the same year the Bath Commission requested that the city furnish funds for enlarging bath no. 1; receiving no response, they again turned to Walters for aid. The following year he donated an additional $15,000 for that purpose.[68]

Walters Bath No. 3 for Negroes opened in December 1905. It had 15 showers and 2 tubs as well as a public laundry; 12 more showers were added in 1907. However, attendance at bath no. 3 was the lowest of any of Baltimore's public baths, and in 1909 the commission arranged for a course of lectures on the value of bathing to be delivered in African-American churches. These efforts apparently did not achieve the desired results, for patrons of bath no. 3 in 1914 numbered 36,466 as opposed to 250,672 for bath no. 1 in the same year. The public laundry of bath no. 3, in contrast, was the most heavily utilized of all the Baltimore public laundries. Although the Bath Commission noted the large patronage, it never stated the obvious conclusion that many of the laundry patrons were washerwomen at work rather than housewives doing their family laundry.[69]

The Baltimore public laundries were well equipped with large washtubs with wringers, hot and cold water, a drying room, and ironing boards and irons. After 1918, playrooms were established in the public laundries where small children could play while their mothers laundered.[70]

In 1910 Henry Walters donated one more bath to the City of Baltimore. Walters Bath No. 4, which opened in April 1911, was located in South Baltimore to serve immigrant East European Jews and Poles. The largest of the Walters baths and including a public comfort station as well as showers, tubs, and laundry, it had cost over $30,000 to construct. Though the bath was sober in design, the Bath Commission stated that an attempt had been made "to give an architectural expression to the exterior, becoming the dignity of the city, and work of a public character."[71]

Baltimore's last municipal bath was constructed by the city itself and opened in 1912. It was probably Baltimore's most elaborate bath, for it was built in an adaptation of Spanish mission style architecture of gray-green stucco with stone trimmings and a heavy canopied cornice covered with glazed green tiles. It was located in a predominantly East European Jewish immigrant area. Henry Walters was prepared to donate a fifth bath to the city and did donate the land and three old buildings on Eastern Avenue in East Baltimore, a section that was home to several immigrant groups. However, this bath was never built, although one of the buildings was remodeled into a small bath with showers (see map 5).[72]

In addition to the supervision of the completion of the Baltimore public bath system and the administration of the existing baths, the Free Public Bath Commission of Baltimore was active in recommending and implementing improvements, innovations, and additions to the existing facilities. Although the city authorities were not usually immediately

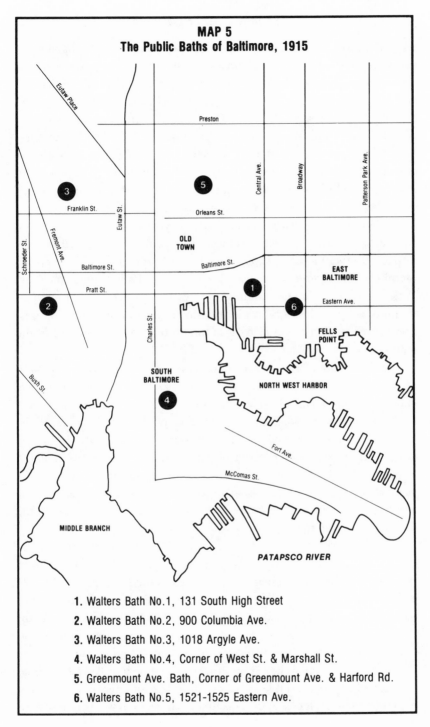

**MAP 5**
**The Public Baths of Baltimore, 1915**

1. Walters Bath No.1, 131 South High Street
2. Walters Bath No.2, 900 Columbia Ave.
3. Walters Bath No.3, 1018 Argyle Ave.
4. Walters Bath No.4, Corner of West St. & Marshall St.
5. Greenmount Ave. Bath, Corner of Greenmount Ave. & Harford Rd.
6. Walters Bath No.5, 1521-1525 Eastern Ave.

responsive to the commission's recommendations, the commission was very persistent in its demands and eventually they were met by the city.

As early as 1903 the Bath Commission, under the leadership of Beadenkopf and Dr. Gichner, had suggested the establishment in the public schools of baths that would be open to the public after school hours. Year after year the commission worked toward this goal until in 1913 the first school bath was constructed. However, because of conflict with the school board this bath was not open to the public until 1916, when the Bath Commission agreed to pay all expenses in connection with its operation. By 1924, shower baths were in operation in eleven schools after school hours with a total attendance for that year of 323,061.[73]

In 1904 the Bath Commission began to urge that the city build public restrooms, and in 1906, $20,000 was appropriated for this purpose. Members of the commission visited Washington, Philadelphia, and New York City to study similar buildings, and Baltimore's first public comfort station was opened in 1908 under the supervision of the Bath Commission. Three more were built by 1915 in addition to those located in the bathhouses.[74]

The Bath Commission also did not ignore outdoor recreational bathing facilities, although it was opposed to the location of swimming pools in the year-round baths. Besides continually encouraging the city to build outdoor swimming pools in every section of the city because of the increasing pollution of the beach baths, the commission also urged the city to buy beach-front property for recreational use in less polluted sections of the waterfront. It also instituted swimming lessons at the beaches and swimming pools in 1909. In 1918, however, the outdoor baths and swimming pools were transferred from the jurisdiction of the Bath Commission to the park board.[75]

An innovation in the municipal bath movement introduced by the Baltimore Bath Commission was the portable shower bath. Thomas Beadenkopf was the originator of this idea, which was inspired by an article in the magazine *Charities and the Commons* that suggested public baths should open their water mains in the summer to offer spray baths to children. Beadenkopf carried this suggestion one step further and "visualized a gospel tent which could be quickly rigged up close to a city fire plug, and in which shower equipment could be installed." Baltimore established its first portable shower bath in the summer of 1908. A tent with four showers, it cost $150. This first portable bath was such a success that new portable baths were designed with light wooden framework, galvanized iron sides and partitions, and a wooden floor. A wooden lean-to on the side contained a coal stove which heated water for a 75–100-gallon water tank. It could be disassembled and moved by two men. These portable baths cost between $600 and $650 to construct and about $30 per week to maintain. In 1910 Baltimore was operating six of these portable baths (one for African Americans) and they were kept open year-round. However, once the school baths were opened to the public, the portable baths were no longer necessary and were discontinued after 1923.[76]

The Free Public Bath Commission of Baltimore, like the Public Baths Association of Philadelphia, was also active in the national and international municipal bath movements. Some of its members played an important part in the founding of the American Association for Promoting Hygiene and Public Baths. Doctor Joseph Gichner served as president of the association and both he and Beadenkopf served as vice-presidents. Beadenkopf was selected by the City of Baltimore to attend the International Conference on Public Baths and School Baths held in 1912 in the Netherlands, where he spoke on Baltimore's portable baths. In addition to being involved in these formal activities, members of the Bath Commission lectured informally on the subject in various cities in the United States and Europe. The Bath Commission received frequent inquiries from all over the United States and even one from Tientsin, China.[77]

Baltimore's baths enjoyed higher patronage than those of most cities that had baths for cleanliness only without recreational facilities. Attendance grew steadily from 48,827 in 1900, the year Walters Bath No. 1 was opened, to a peak of 753,899 in 1914. After this, patronage at the public baths began to decline slowly, leveling off at about 600,000 during the 1920s, although the Bath Commission was able to report increases by including the number of showers taken in the school baths in the total. The Bath Commission attributed the decline in use of the public baths to the extension of Baltimore's sewer system and the more general installation of bathtubs in homes.[78]

The net expense of maintaining and operating Baltimore's bath system was, like that for Philadelphia's, very modest because the small fees charged for the use of the baths and laundries helped to defray operating costs. In 1912, with all Baltimore's five permanent baths (as well as six portable baths) in operation, the net expense was $24,675.[79]

Baltimore's public bath movement was unique, however, in its combined private-public character and like Philadelphia's in the sustained interest of its bath reformers in the bath system. Although Henry Walters donated all the baths except one, the municipal government operated them. Thomas Beadenkopf advocated public baths from the beginning, served on the Bath Commission from its inception, and was superintendent of the baths until his death in 1915. Eugene Levering was president of the commission from 1895 until his death in 1928, and Dr. Mary Sherwood served on the commission for over twenty-five years.

Baltimore's municipal baths became the target of an economy drive in the 1950s as their patronage dwindled and the expense of maintaining them rose (the maintenance appropriation for the baths in 1959 was $291,676). As a result, the baths were closed in 1960.[80]

In Philadelphia and Baltimore, private philanthropy provided public bath systems when the municipal governments of these cities failed to do so. As we have seen, bath advocates urged wealthy individuals to donate baths to their cities and some did. Andrew Carnegie in *The Gospel of Wealth* favored such gifts as libraries, parks, concert halls, museums, and baths which would serve the able and industrious as "ladders upon which the aspiring can rise." Even Washington Gladden, before his concern with "tainted wealth," included public baths as suitable projects for wealthy benefactors. Public baths, like museums and libraries, would extend to the city's poor some of the amenities of urban life but, unlike museums and libraries, were located in poor neighborhoods, thus conforming to the progressive ideal of neighborhood level reform. The upper class members of Philadelphia's Public Baths Association and Henry Walters were providing their cities with facilities that they felt all cities should provide for the health and moral well-being of their poorer citizens. In doing so they improved the status of their cities as civic communities and brought them closer to the urban ideal in the Progressive Era.[81]

Having achieved success in the five cities under discussion as well as in other cities throughout the United States, either through municipal action or through private philanthropy, the bath reformers in 1912 formally organized themselves in a national association.

# 6

## The American Association for Promoting Hygiene and Public Baths

Health Is Wealth

With "Health Is Wealth" as their official motto, the bath reformers organized the American Association for Promoting Hygiene and Public Baths in New York City in May 1912, approximately a decade after the public bath movement in the United States had reached its peak. Most American cities by 1912 had either completed or were near completion of their bath systems. The official organization of the bath movement, however, only institutionalized the informal network of bath reformers that had existed since the 1890s.[1]

At the heart of this network were Simon Baruch and the New York AICP's People's Baths, which opened in 1891. Boston's Public Bath Commission, Gertrude Gail Wellington of Chicago's Municipal Order League, and the Public Baths Association of Philadelphia all made pilgrimages to New York to inspect the People's Baths and confer with Baruch. As the network widened, Mayor Josiah Quincy of Boston and Franklin J. Kirkbride of Philadelphia spoke in Baltimore on the necessity of public baths. Reverend Thomas Beadenkopf of the Baltimore Bath Commission journeyed to Philadelphia, New York City, Boston, and Chicago to survey their bath systems before the commission made its recommendations to Henry Walters. Not only did the bath proponents from cities that had bath systems offer their expertise to their counterparts from other cities planning to set up such systems, but bath reformers journeyed to inspect each other's bath systems, share information, and compare their progress.[2]

The bath reformers also made extensive use of newspapers and magazines to publicize the need for public baths and to disseminate the accomplishments of the public bath movement. Local newspapers not only published feature articles on the bath systems of their own cities but also reported on those of other cities. In their editorial pages they repeatedly urged that their cities build adequate bath systems. Between 1895 and 1915, magazines concerned with the social issues of the day and urban problems, such as *Survey, Outlook, Charities, American City, Municipal Affairs,* and the *Annals,* published many articles on public baths. Bath reformers, such as Josiah Quincy and Franklin B. Kirkbride, frequently contributed to these publications during the time that they were active in the movement.[3]

The bath reformers decided to formalize their informal network when the International Conference on Public and School Baths was announced to meet in the Netherlands in August 1912. Several European countries had national public baths associations, and American bath advocates set up a similar association so they could formally select delegates to attend the conference.

The Reverend Thomas Beadenkopf, superintendent of Baltimore's public baths, suggested the organizational meeting that met in New York City in May 1912. Some thirty-five to forty people attended this meeting, including the superintendents of the public bath systems of Boston, Manhattan, Brooklyn, Philadelphia, and Pittsburgh. Simon Baruch was elected president and Beadenkopf vice-president of the new association. The treasurer was August Windolph, a member of the architectural firm Werner and Windolph, which specialized in planning public baths. The recording secretary was Jennie Wells Wentworth, who was a special investigator in Manhattan's Department of Public Works (which had jurisdiction over the borough's municipal baths). Doctor William Henry Hale, who was superintendent of Brooklyn's municipal baths, was elected permanent secretary.[4]

The directors of the association included W. L. Ross, H. C. McGrath, and Frank L. Hines, superintendents of the Philadelphia, Boston, and Manhattan bath systems, respectively, and members of the bath commissions of Baltimore and Newark. Persons active in public health, such as Wallace A. Manheimer, a bacteriologist from the New York City Department of Health and the Columbia University faculty, and Mary L. Jacobson, a member of the Newark, New Jersey, public bath improvement association, were also directors.[5]

The leadership of the American Association for Promoting Hygiene and Public Baths was, therefore, in the beginning a combination of bath reformers, like Beadenkopf and Baruch, who had actively advocated the cause of public baths since the 1890s, and persons who had not originally been bath advocates but who were professionals who administered and operated municipal bath systems or were involved in public health work. As with many other social reforms in the Progressive Era the public bath movement became increasingly professionalized. The formation of the association was a symbol of this transformation from reform to scientific management of the institutions that the reformers had advocated.[6]

As time went on, the professional aspect of the association became more pronounced as the original bath advocates died. Beadenkopf, who died in 1915, was replaced as vice-president by Dr. Joseph Gichner, a member of the Free Public Bath Commission of Baltimore. When Baruch died in 1921, his successor as president was Dr. Thomas Darlington, professor of anatomy at the New York College of Dentistry and former commissioner of health of New York City. Gichner became president upon Darlington's resignation in 1928.[7]

The increasing professionalism of the association was reflected also in its new members, who in the 1920s were public baths personnel, public health officers (especially sanitary engineers, bacteriologists, and chemists), architects, and public recreation personnel. This professionalization occurred as a matter of course once a reform was in place and required administration and supervision. In the case of public baths it may have been more pronounced because by the 1920s the need for them was declining and there was little impetus to build more.[8]

The American Association for Promoting Hygiene and Public Baths, like the municipal bath movement itself, was confined mostly to the northeastern and middle Atlantic states. At the first meeting in 1912, Pittsburgh was the westernmost city represented and Baltimore was the southernmost. The officers, too, were with rare exceptions either from New York or Baltimore and the bath leaders of these two cities dominated the association. By 1921, however, the association had a somewhat more national character. The board of directors included Chicago's commissioner of health (who had jurisdiction over that city's municipal bath system), the chief sanitary engineer of the Florida State Board of Health, and a director from Berkeley, California, whose occupation cannot be determined. The annual conferences of the association were always held in the East, with Baltimore and New York as the most common host cities. Richmond, Virginia; Brookline, Massachusetts; Newark and Jersey City, New Jersey; and Saratoga Springs and Buffalo, New York, also hosted annual conferences. Pittsburgh was the westernmost city to serve as a conference site; Boston, Philadelphia, and Chicago never did.[9]

The first official action of the American Association for Promoting Hygiene and Public Baths was to select two of its members to attend the International Conference on Public and School Baths in August 1912. The members selected were William Henry Hale, superintendent of the Brooklyn baths, and William Paul Gerhard, a sanitary engineer and frequent author on the subject of public baths, also from Brooklyn. Two other Americans also attended this conference: Thomas Beadenkopf, who was sent by the City of Baltimore, and Mrs. Tunis Bergen, a Brooklyn bath advocate.[10]

The three men delivered papers at the conference. Hale spoke on "The Public Baths of New York City," Gerhard on "The Progress of the Public Bath Movement in the United States," and Beadenkopf on "The Portable Baths of Baltimore," illustrated with lantern slides. The topics of other papers included school baths, baths in industry, swimming baths, the physiology of bathing, and reports on the progress of the public bath movement in twelve countries. In addition the International Association for Public Baths and Cleanliness was organized with permanent offices at The Hague and with a membership list of over 600 names, including the four Americans who attended the conference as well as Simon Baruch, who did not attend.[11]

Several American organizations sent exhibits to the Public Baths Exposition sponsored by the international conference. These groups included the city of New York, the New York AICP, the New York City departments of Public Education and Public Health, the Public Baths Association of Philadelphia, and the Free Public Bath Commission of Baltimore.[12]

At the end of the international conference a series of resolutions were passed endorsing the shower bath as the most effective means of attaining personal cleanliness, urging all cities and schools to maintain shower baths, recommending that regular baths become part of the school cur-

riculum, and recommending that swimming pools and swimming in-
structions be a supplemental part of public bath systems. Plans were
made for the international association to hold biennial meetings, the next
one to be held in Brussels in August 1914. The activities of the international association were, however, disrupted by World War I and did not
resume until the 1920s. William Gerhard continued to play an active role
in the association, and the American Association for Promoting Hygiene
and Public Baths from time to time published news of its activities. In
1927 the American association formally joined the international association and began to urge the calling of another international conference to
meet in New York City, but there is no evidence that this conference ever
materialized.[13]

After its founding in 1912, the American Association for Promoting
Hygiene and Public Baths held yearly meetings at which members
elected officers and toured the bath facilities of the host city, and some
members delivered papers. Beginning in 1916 the association began to
publish the minutes of its annual meetings and the papers read at the
meetings. At the outset, these were published in *Proceedings,* but in 1918
and thereafter they were published as the *Journal of the American Association
for Promoting Hygiene and Public Baths.*[14]

Until the early 1920s the *Journal* articles were in the main concerned
with public baths and bore such titles as "Campaign Work for Promoting
Public Baths," "Portable Bath Houses," and "Model Bath Houses and
Recreation Centers." Gradually, the emphasis in the *Journal* moved away
from public baths to several other areas of more professional interest.
One of these areas was swimming pools, and many articles were written
on the subject, especially on technical aspects such as the purification of
water in swimming pools by various methods. The *Journal* also began to
print, on a regular basis, state rules and regulations regarding the operation and maintenance of public swimming pools. Other areas of concentration were public health, including such topics as visiting nurses,
rural health work and garbage disposal, and public recreation. In these
aspects the association cooperated with the American Public Health
Assocation and the American Physical Education Association. Advertisements in the *Journal* also reflected these changes in emphasis from public
bath equipment to swimming pool needs.[15]

After Simon Baruch's death in 1921, the American Association for
Promoting Hygiene and Public Baths began to hold yearly memorial

services in honor of Baruch at New York City's Rivington Street Bath, which was renamed in his honor. These memorial services were usually fairly elaborate with musical selections by the Department of Sanitation Band, several speeches by members of the association, the placement of a wreath on the Baruch memorial tablet, and the distribution of candy to the children present by the Baruch family. After the memorial service the association generally held its annual business meeting, which now was separate from the annual conference.[16]

In the 1920s the association voted honorary memberships to a number of prominent individuals, including William G. McAdoo and Andrew Mellon. Honorary membership was also extended to Eugene Levering, chairman of the Baltimore Bath Commission; the surgeon-generals of the United States Public Health Service and of the Army and Navy; various national public baths associations, including those of Germany, the Netherlands, and Norway; and the International Association for Public Baths and Cleanliness.[17]

Although the American Association for Promoting Hygiene and Public Baths held its annual business meetings in New York City and continued to publish its *Journal* from 1926 to 1929, no annual conferences were held during this period. The association appears to have ceased its activities, including the publication of the *Journal,* in the early 1930s.[18]

Thus, in 1912 the municipal bath movement, after two decades of agitation and the realization of most of its demands, formally organized itself on a national scale. In the long run, however, the American Association for Promoting Hygiene and Public Baths was not really an organization of reformers who worked for the further extension of the municipal bath movement in the United States (although this was their purpose in the beginning), but rather a professional organization of those responsible for the maintenance and operation of existing public bath systems.

# 7

## The Gospel of Cleanliness

The greatest justification for the public bath is its educational influence. It may make people now poorly housed more insistent upon that part of housing reform which will give them, eventually, bath equipment in the home.

—DONALD B. ARMSTRONG

By 1914, when these words were written, the public bath movement had peaked and it had become obvious to the bath reformers that patronage of the baths did not meet their expectations. Yet some of them had come to realize that, although many of the great unwashed had not been converted into users of public baths, they were becoming converted to the gospel of personal cleanliness.

In spite of this changing focus, the actual process of public bath reform on the local level provides interesting historical insights. Its international character, its diverse leadership, the variety of responses in the cities considered, the combination of public and private provision of public baths, and the motivations of its reformers all reveal the complexities of urban social reform and the difficulties inherent in generalizing about a reform which had its origins in the mid-nineteenth century and achieved success during the Progressive Era.

The public bath movement had its genesis in both the rising American concern for cleanliness in the mid-nineteenth century and the example of the public baths of European cities. Like the settlement house leaders, public bath proponents were influenced by English models, but they were also very impressed by Continental practices. Both Simon Baruch of New York and Thomas M. Beadenkopf of Baltimore visited German public baths and urged that American cities base their bath systems on

German models. The movement itself was international and, as we have seen, American bath proponents were also active in the organization of the International Association for Public Baths and Cleanliness and continued to participate during the 1920s.

The leadership of the public bath movement illustrates the diverse character of urban progressive reformers, who were in this case united by this single issue. One charitable organization, the New York Association for Improving the Condition of the Poor, was a consistent advocate of public baths and built the very influential prototype of the People's Baths. In Philadelphia the Public Baths Association, a private charitable organization, was responsible for the only year-round baths located in that city. Individual philanthropists also presented public baths to their cities, as bath advocates urged them to do. Henry Walters of Baltimore was the leading donor, but Pittsburgh, Richmond (Virginia), New York City, and San Francisco also were presented with public baths by wealthy citizens.[1]

Some politicians were leaders in the bath movement or lent it strong support. Although the bath movement in New York City seems at first to be a simple case of reformers versus the bosses of Tammany Hall and although reform mayors Strong and Low were its firmest supporters, later Tammany leaders endorsed the movement. In Boston the strongest supporters of public baths were some of its mayors: the patrician reformer Josiah Quincy and the Irish machine politicians John Fitzgerald and James Michael Curley.

Physicians, because of their interest in public health, also were in the vanguard of the movement and its foremost leader was Dr. Simon Baruch of New York City. In Chicago, a group of women physicians, leaders of the Free Bath and Sanitary League supported by a network of women reformers, convinced the municipal government to build that city's first public baths. Women also served as members of the bath commissions of Boston and Baltimore, and a woman was instrumental in the organization of the Public Baths Association of Philadelphia. Asserting their role as "municipal housekeepers," these women found themselves moving naturally from the private sphere into the public sphere.

Settlement house leaders male and female, such as Robert Woods in Boston and Jane Addams and Mary McDowell in Chicago, were strong supporters of public baths which would improve the lives of their poor neighbors. Settlement houses themselves often maintained a few shower baths, and they cooperated fully with the bath reformers of their cities by organizing their neighbors to campaign for baths and putting pressure on city governments. With the exception of Woods, however, public baths were not in the forefront of reforms that settlement house leaders advocated.

Businessmen as a group were often interested in political and economic reform in their cities but were seldom found in the ranks of urban social reformers. Nevertheless, they were very active in the public bath movement as leaders and philanthropists. Eugene Levering, a Baltimore banker, headed its Public Bath Commission for over thirty years, and the members of the Public Baths Association of Philadelphia were some of that city's leading businessmen. Robert Wiebe maintained that "the only important contribution which businessmen made to the social welfare movement came as a by-product of their zeal for civic improvement. As they scrubbed and polished their cities, some did assist in improving local housing and health codes."[2] However, the businessmen who were bath reformers were primarily interested in providing an essential city service that would help the poorer citizens of their cities and safeguard the public health. Beautifying or improving the appearance of their cities was of secondary importance to them in this case. Additionally, almost all the businessmen involved in the public bath movement were also active in a variety of other charitable activities.

The leaders of the public bath movement were for the most part middle and upper class, native-born Protestant Americans educated at prestigious colleges. Mostly from affluent families, many were wealthy in their own right. They were professionals and businessmen; one, Thomas K. Beadenkopf, was a Congregational minister. Yet the movement did have an interethnic character. Simon Baruch was both an immigrant and a Jew; and the chairman of Boston's Bath Commission, its Irish bosses, and Baltimore's Henry Walters were Catholics. Although labor leaders were represented on the mayors' committees on public baths in New York and Boston, they were only peripherally interested in the cause and were not important advocates. Among the great unwashed there was little interest or enthusiasm. With the exception of a few public meetings in New York City and support rallied by settlement house workers in Boston and Chicago, there was no mass advocacy in slum neighborhoods for public baths. This was truly a reform offered from above.

By the turn of the century there was general agreement that it was the responsibility of city governments to provide public baths for the poor. However, because this was local reform, it was achieved in a variety of ways in the cities under consideration. Basically the decision of whether, when, and how to build public baths was political, and bath reformers had to deal with the political conditions in each of their cities to achieve their objective. New York City, after a decade of delay, built the most elaborate and expensive bath system in the country. Boston combined most of its baths with recreational facilities and thereby attracted the most satisfactory patronage. Chicago came closest to the bath reformers' ideal by building many modest and utilitarian baths in slum neighborhoods. In Philadelphia and Baltimore, where the municipal governments were slow to comply, private charity assumed responsibility. In Baltimore, once the baths were built and presented to the city, it assumed administration of them and paid the operating expenses. In all these cities, however, once the bath system was an operating reality, the movement, like much of the social reform of the Progressive Era, of necessity became professionalized and bureaucratized.

The motivation of the public bath reformers is complex. Certainly they were interested in social control, that is, they were attempting to impose middle- or upper-class standards of behavior on the lower classes and to increase the order and stability of their rapidly changing cities.[3] But, in advocating the cleanliness of the poor, they were not coercive. They sought conformity by persuasion and were confident that, once provided with bathing facilities, the poor would change their ways. They maintained that not only would the poor be clean, but also their moral character would be enhanced, and slum conditions would be improved. For the bath reformers, as for other Americans, personal cleanliness had assumed a symbolic meaning; it stood for respectability, admission to the middle class, and citizenship in the urban community.

Cleanliness also had assumed symbolic importance in the process of Americanization and assimilation of immigrants, who comprised more than one-third of the population of three of the cities under discussion. Immigrants also constituted the majority of slum dwellers. Conforming to American standards of cleanliness was a crucial step on the road to acculturation and, as we have seen, most public baths were located in immigrant neighborhoods. Even though public bath advocates claimed that these institutions were to serve the poor, the people they served were mostly poor immigrants.

Public baths would also, bath proponents believed, provide a measure of social justice or redress some of the inequities of urban life. As Josiah Quincy maintained, municipal governments must "secure in some measure the enjoyment by all, not, indeed, of an impossible equality of social opportunity, but of a certain minimum of elementary social advantages."[4] The bath reformers did not seek to supply the poor with the private bathrooms in their homes which they enjoyed, but instead would build public baths. This is in contrast to European public baths, which served both the poor and the middle class (in separate sections, to be sure).

American bath reformers stressed the utilitarian function of public baths. The short time allotted for bathing and the control of the water temperature communicated the primacy of the cleanliness function. Although many public baths included recreational facilities such as swimming pools and gymnasiums, reformers saw them as means of improving the health and physical fitness of the poor and of attracting them to the baths. The strict separation of the sexes was meant to ensure that these public baths would have none of the unsavory connotations of those of the past (or the future). Bath advocates almost never mentioned the pleasurable and sensual aspects of bathing, such as rejuvenation, invigoration, or relaxation. They wanted the poor to be clean but seemingly did not want them to enjoy it too much.[5]

The public bath movement may represent a case of class and ethnic conflict between middle- and upper-class reformers and the objects of their reform. While there is almost no record of the reactions of the poor to the public baths, they did use them, although not in the numbers expected by the reformers.[6] The statistics show that the baths were utilized to their capacity only on the hottest summer days and attendance was very low in the winter, except where the baths were connected to recreational facilities, as they were in Boston. An incident in New York City in which bath patrons bribed bath attendants so they could bathe for as long as they liked, indicates resistance to the no-nonsense approach to bathing. Also in New York City, a "small scale riot" occurred during a heat wave in the summer of 1906, when 5,000 persons waiting to bathe at the Rivington Street Bath were told that it was closing. The police had to intervene to restore order. It seems obvious that the bath patrons used the public baths for their own purposes, not just to be clean but also for relaxation and relief from summer heat.[7]

Paradoxically, although the appearance of some public baths, such as the inexpensive, modest baths of Chicago, conveyed their utilitarian cleanliness function, others were architecturally distinguished and even luxurious. New York's neo-Roman East 23rd Street Bath (now the Asser Levy Bath) with its marble bath cubicles and marble swimming pool decorated with a brass lion's head fountain, Boston's Dover Street Bath with its terrazzo mosaic floors and marble walls and staircases, and its North Bennet Street Bath and Gymnasium with its architecture adapted from the Villa Medici in Rome provided very pleasant surroundings for bathing. Although the bath reformers can be criticized for not demanding for the poor the same private baths in their homes which they enjoyed and for not making allowances for the pleasurable aspects of bathing, some of the public baths were, as Josiah Quincy maintained, "architectural monument[s] of the city" and did "raise the whole idea of public bathing to a high and dignified plane."[8]

Certainly the fact that cities and philanthropists provided public baths for the poor and the fact that some of these baths were expensive and imposing, communicated the idea that personal cleanliness was an important aspect of full membership in the communities in which they lived. These bathhouses were tangible witness to the exhortations of the bath reformers on the significance of cleanliness. And in fact cleanliness was critical for those who were seeking better employment, and for social acceptance in public places and in schools, in other words, for social and economic mobility. The bath reformers seemed to have considered that the main patrons of public baths would be workingmen and transients in that they invariably provided more showers for men and boys than for women and girls or, as in Chicago, opened the public baths to women and girls two days per week and to men and boys the rest of the time. The percentage of women bathers ranged from a low of about 10 percent in Philadelphia to a high of about 30 percent in Boston. Bath reformers attributed the lack of female patrons to various causes ranging from modesty, timidity, and the pressures of home duties to the difficulty in drying their hair.[9]

Bath reformers made a strenuous attempt to convert schoolchildren to the gospel of cleanliness, most especially by providing showers in the public schools but also by publicizing nearby baths in local schools. Public schools also did their part by scheduling weekly shower baths for each student during the school day in schools that had showers, and by stressing the importance of personal cleanliness in health and hygiene curricula at the turn of the century and well into the twentieth century.[10]

The educational effect of the public bath movement was its most lasting legacy. The poor did not reject the gospel of cleanliness, although they did not use the public baths to the extent that the bath reformers expected. What they wanted and what they eventually got was what the middle-class reformers already had—baths in their own homes.[11]

David Glassberg has seen the provision of public baths as a stopgap measure to ensure the cleanliness of the poor until they had bathing facilities in their own homes. The bath reformers and the municipal governments and philanthropists who built public baths, however, considered them to be permanent institutions. But by the time that the bath movement reached its peak (1900–10), standards in housing for the poor had begun to change, especially in the matter of the provision of bathrooms. As has been noted, tenement house laws passed around 1900 generally required that apartments include a separate toilet and many builders included a bathtub as well. New tenements after this time almost always included private bathrooms, which became more inexpensive with the invention (in 1916) and mass production of the one-piece galvanized, enameled bathtub. More and more the poor had bathtubs in their homes. A 1917–18 study of Philadelphia workingmen's standard of living reported that 86.2 percent had bathtubs in their homes and considered a "fair standard of housing to include a bathroom with toilet, washstand and tub." The United States Bureau of Labor studied the housing conditions of the poor in twenty cities in 1918–19 and reported that over one-half the families had baths. Their report also asserted that "it is felt that a housing standard to provide health and decency must include a complete bathroom with toilet."[12]

During the 1920s the number of the urban poor who had private bathrooms continued to increase. Even among the poorest the majority had bathrooms. A 1928–32 study of 113 Chicago households on relief found that only 18 were without bathrooms. In 1934 during the Great Depression, a survey of New York City dwelling units uncovered only 11.4 percent without bathtubs or showers. As the federal government began to build low income housing during the New Deal, the Public Works Administration housing standards required a private bathroom in each apartment. Cities continued to operate their public bath systems during this time to serve this small minority without bathing facilities in their homes.[13]

Another factor that the bath reformers did not consider was the changing nature of urban neighborhoods. As has been pointed out, in New York two public baths were constructed in what were then poor immigrant neighborhoods on the now exclusive Upper East Side. By the 1920s, the East 54th Street Bath was neighbor to the luxurious apartment buildings on Sutton Place; twenty years later the East 76th Street Bath met a similar fate. In other cities similar transformations occurred, although some neighborhoods where baths were located remain slums.

In the two decades after World War II almost all urban dwellers acquired private bathrooms in their homes, and cities gradually closed down their bath systems as they became an expensive and virtually obsolete service. The gospel of cleanliness has become a basic tenet of American life, but it is the private bathroom, growing ever more elaborate and luxurious, and not the public bath that is the bath reformers' monument.

# Appendix I

## New York State
## Public Bath Law of 1892
## Chapter 473

*Section 1.*    It shall be lawful for any city, village or town to establish free public baths. Any city, village or town may loan its credit or make appropriations of its funds for the purpose of establishing free public baths.

*Section 2.*    This act shall take effect immediately.[1]

---

1. Frank Tucker, "Public Baths," in Robert W. DeForest and Lawrence Veiller, eds., *The Tenement House Problem* (New York, Macmillan, 1903), 2:50.

# Appendix II

## New York State
## Public Bath Law of 1895
## Chapter 351

*Section 1.*    All cities of the first and second class shall establish and maintain such number of public baths as the local Board of Health may determine to be necessary; each bath shall be kept open not less than fourteen hours for each day, and both hot and cold water shall be provided. The erection and maintenance of river or ocean baths shall not be deemed a compliance with the requirements of this section. Any city, village or town having less than 50,000 inhabitants may establish and maintain free public baths, and any city, village or town may loan its credit or may appropriate its funds for the purpose of establishing such free public baths.

*Section 2.*    This act shall take effect immediately.[1]

---

1. Tucker, "Public Baths," 42.

# Appendix III

## New York State Public Bath Law of 1896 Chapter 122

*Section 1.*  The Commissioner of Public Works in the City of New York, with the consent and approval of the Board of Estimate and Apportionment of said city, expressed as hereinafter provided, is hereby authorized and empowered to erect such and so many buildings for Free Public Baths, and such and so many structures for the promotion of public comfort within said City of New York as in the opinion of said commissioner of Public Works and said Board of Estimate and Apportionment shall be necessary and proper.

*Section 2.*  Before proceeding to erect or construct any building or structure as authorized by the last preceding section the said Commissioner of Public Works may, from time to time, present to the said Board of Estimate and Apportionment a statement from any work proposed to be done, with plans and specifications therefor, and an estimate of the proximate probable cost therefor, whereupon the said Board of Estimate and Apportionment may, by resolution authorize said work to be done wholly or in part, and may approve of the plans and specifications therefor, or may return the same to said Commissioner of Public Works for modification or alteration, whereupon said Commissioner of Public Works shall resubmit said plans and specifications, and after having modified or altered the same shall again submit them to said Board of Estimate and Apportionment, who may then approve the same or again return them to the said Commissioner of Public Works for further modification or alteration and said plans and specifications may be so returned to said Commissioner of Public Works and resubmitted to said Board of Estimate and Apportionment until the said Board of Estimate and Apportionment shall, by resolution, approve said plans and specifications and authorize the work to be proceeded with accordingly.

*Section 3.*  When any work provided for by this act shall have been authorized and the plans and specifications therefor approved by the Board of Estimate and Apportionment the said Commissioner of Public Works shall proceed to execute and carry out said work, which shall be done by contract, made at public letting to the lowest bidder, pursuant to the general provision of law and ordinances regulating the letting, execution and performance of public contracts in the City of New York. The Commissioner of Public Works, with the approval of the Board of Estimate and Apportionment first had and obtained, is hereby authorized and empowered, with the consent in writing of the contractor and his sureties, to alter any plans, and the terms and specifications of any contract entered into by the authority of this act, provided that such alteration shall in no case involve or require an increased expense greater than five per centum of the whole expenditure provided for in said contract.

**Section 4.**    The Commissioner of Public Works is authorized and empowered with the consent and approval of the Board of Estimate and Apportionment to locate any or all of the structures for the promotion of public comfort to be erected under the authority of this act to be so erected in any public park of the City of New York, and for that purpose the Commissioner of Public Parks shall permit the said Commissioner of Public Works, his officers and agents and the contractors to enter upon said park or parks and therein to perform the work so authorized. Any such structure which may be erected in any public park of said city shall, after its erection and completion, be under the care, custody and control of the Department of Public Parks in said City, who are hereby authorized and empowered to make proper and necessary rules for the use and management thereof.

**Section 5.**    For the purpose of carrying out the work authorized by this act, including compensation of any architect or architects employed by the said Commissioner of Public Works to prepare plans and specifications and to supervise the work done thereunder, and of any architect employed by the Board of Estimate and Apportionment to examine any plans and specifications, and including also the cost of such furniture and fixtures for any building hereby authorized as shall be approved and consented to by the Board of Estimate and Apportionment, the Comptroller of the City of New York is hereby directed, from time to time, when thereto directed by the Board of Estimate and Apportionment, to issue consolidated stock of the City of New York in the manner now provided by law to an amount not exceeding in the aggregate the sum of two hundred thousand dollars.

**Section 6.**    This act shall take effect immediately.[1]

---

1. Tucker, "Public Baths," 46–47.

# Appendix IV

## Public Bath Law of Massachusetts

This law was first enacted in 1874 and was included as sections 20 and 21 of Chapter 25 in the Revised Laws of 1902.

*Section 20.* A town which accepts the provisions of this and the following section, or had accepted the corresponding provisions of earlier laws, by a two-thirds vote at an annual meeting, may purchase or lease lands, and erect, alter, enlarge, repair and improve buildings for public baths and washhouses, either with or without open drying grounds, and may make open bathing places, provide them with the requisite furniture, fittings and conveniences, provide instruction in swimming, and may raise and appropriate money therefor.

*Section 21.* Such towns may establish rates for the use of such baths and washhouses, and appoint officers therefor, and may make by-laws for the government of such officers, and authorize them to make regulations for the management thereof and for the use thereof by non-residents of said town.[1]

---

1. G. W. W. Hanger, "Public Baths in the United States," in U.S. Department of Commerce and Labor, *Bulletin of the Bureau of Labor* 9 (Washington, D.C.: Government Printing Office, 1904), 1251.

# Notes

## Introduction

1   U.S. Census Office, *12th Census of the United States: 1900 Population* (Washington, D.C.: Government Printing Office, 1903), 1:lxix.

## Chapter 1

1   Jacob A. Riis, *How the Other Half Lives: Studies Among the Tenements of New York* (n.p.: Telegraph Books, 1985, orig. pub. 1890), 83–84.

2   U.S. Census Office, J. D. B. DeBow, *Statistical View of the United States: Compendium of the Seventh Census* (Washington, D.C.: A. O. P. Nicholson, 1854), 192; U.S. Bureau of the Census, *Historical Statistics of the United States, Colonial Times to 1970,* Bicentennial Edition (Washington, D.C.: Government Printing Office, 1975), 1:106. For a summary and analysis of urban reform in the nineteenth century, see Paul Boyer, *Urban Masses and Moral Order in America, 1820–1920* (Cambridge, Mass.: Harvard University Press, 1978), chaps. 1–12.

3   William Paul Gerhard, *Modern Baths and Bath Houses* (New York: John Wiley & Sons, 1908), 1–4; Simon Baruch, *A Plea for Public Baths, together with an Inexpensive Method for Their Hygienic Utilization,* reprint from the *Dietetic Gazette,* May 1891, 7–8, 11–12; A. G. Varron, "Hygiene in the Medieval City," *Ciba Symposium* 1 (Oct. 1939), 213; Lynn Thorndike, "Sanitation, Baths and Street-cleaning in the Middle Ages and the Renaissance," *Speculum* 3 (1928), 196–99; Philippe Braunstein, "Toward Intimacy: The Fourteenth and Fifteenth Centuries," in Georges Duby, ed., *A History of Private Life, vol. 2: Revelations of the Medieval World,* trans. by Arthur Goldhammer (Cambridge and London: Belknap Press of Harvard University, 1988), 600–609; George Rosen, *A History of Public Health* (New York: MD Publications, 1958), 79; Siegfried Giedion, *Mechanization Takes Command* (New York: Oxford University Press, 1948), 652–54.

4   Varron, 214; George Ryley Scott, *The Story of Baths and Bathing* (London:

T. Werner Laurie, 1939), 152; Lawrence Wright, *Clean and Decent: The Fascinating History of the Bath-room and the Water Closet* (London and Boston: Routledge and Kegan Paul, 1966), 98–99; Harold Donaldson Eberlein, "When Society First Took a Bath," *Pennsylvania Magazine of History and Biography* 67 (Jan. 1943), 39–40; Agnes Campbell, *Report on Public Baths and Wash-houses in the United Kingdom* (Edinburgh: T. & A. Constable, 1918), 2.

5  Rosen, 219; Edward H. Gibson, III, "Baths and Washhouses in the English Public Health Agitation 1839–48," *Journal of the History of Medicine and Allied Sciences* 9 (Oct. 1954), 391–93; on rising middle-class standards of cleanliness in England and Germany, see Lenore Davidoff and Catherine Hall, *Family Fortunes: Men and Women of the English Middle Class, 1780–1850* (London: Hutchinson, 1987), 382–83, and Brian K. Ladd, "Public Baths and Civic Improvement in Nineteenth-Century German Cities," *Journal of Urban History* 14 (May 1988), 374–77.

6  Edward Mussey Hartwell, "Public Baths in Europe," in Charles H. Verrill, ed., *Monographs on Social Economics,* No. 6 (Washington, D.C.: U.S. Department of Labor Exhibit, Pan-American Exposition, 1901), 2; Scott, 157; Rosen, 219; Arthur Ashpitel and John Whichcord, *Baths and Wash-houses* (London: T. T. Richards, 1853), 35; Gibson, 396–403.

7  Robert Owen Allsop, *Public Baths and Wash-houses* (London: E. & F. N. Spon, 1894), 4–8; Alfred W. S. Cross, *Public Baths and Wash-houses* (London: B. T. Botsford, 1906), 233–45.

8  Hartwell, 5, 8, 10.

9  Campbell, 39; Allsop, 83–84.

10  Milo Ray Maltbie, "Public Baths," *Municipal Affairs* 2 (Dec. 1898), 687.

11  Alfred Martin, "On Bathing," *Ciba Symposia* 1 (Aug. 1939), 147–48; Hartwell, 22–23, 42; Giedion, 677–78; Baruch, *Plea for Public Baths,* 24, 32; for a study of the German public bath movement, see Ladd, 372–93.

12  Hartwell, 46; Giedion, 677; Baruch, *Plea,* 24–32.

13  Maltbie, 687–88; Hartwell, 36.

14  Hartwell, 1. For reference to Japanese baths, see, e.g., *Brooklyn Daily Eagle,* Jan. 29, 1895, and William Paul Gerhard, "People's Baths," *Public Improvements* 1 (Sept. 15, 1899), 192.

15  Carl Bridenbaugh, "Baths and Watering Places of Colonial America," *William and Mary Quarterly,* 3d ser., 3 (Apr. 1946), 152–58, quotations on 171.

16  Ibid., 152, 157–58, 160–63; John Adams, *Works, Diary,* ed. Charles Francis Adams (Boston: Little, Brown, 1850), 2: 264, 268.

17  Eberlein, 39; *Daily Advertiser* (New York), June 5, 1792, quoted in I. N. Phelps Stokes, *The Iconography of Manhattan Island 1648–1909* (New York: Robert H. Dodd, 1928), 5:1289.

18  Eberlein, 48; Bessie Louise Pierce, *A History of Chicago* (New York: Alfred A. Knopf, 1937), 1:201.

19 Eberlein, 39–42, quotation on 42; Bridenbaugh, 175–76.
20 Eberlein, 47–48; Allan Nevins and Milton Halsey Thomas, eds., *The Diary of George Templeton Strong* (New York: Macmillan, 1952), 1:210; Richard L. Bushman and Claudia L. Bushman, "The Early History of Cleanliness in America," *Journal of American History* 74 (Mar. 1988), 1225. Indoor bathing fixtures like these became available to suburbanites from about the 1870s on as water and sewer systems were extended beyond city limits. See Ann Durkin Keating, *Building Chicago: Suburban Developers and the Creation of a Divided Metropolis* (Columbus: Ohio State University Press, 1988), 54–57.
21 Ronald L. Numbers, "Do It Yourself the Sectarian Way," in Judith Walzer Leavitt and Ronald M. Numbers, eds., *Sickness and Health in America: Readings in the History of Medicine and Public Health* (Madison: University of Wisconsin Press, 1978), 91–93; Harry B. Weiss and Howard R. Kemble, *The Great American Water Cure Craze: A History of Hydropathy in the United States* (Trenton, N.J.: Past Times Press, 1967); Marshall Scott Legan, "Hydropathy in America: A Nineteenth Century Panacea," *Bulletin of the History of Medicine* 45 (1971), 267–80. For the importance of hydropathy as a treatment for women's health problems, see Jane B. Donegan, *"Hydropathic Highway to Health": Women and the Water Cure in Antebellum America* (Westport, Conn.: Greenwood Press, 1986), xi–xvi, 3–14, 192–97; and Susan E. Cayleff, *Wash and Be Healed: the Water Cure Movement and Women's Health* (Philadelphia: Temple University Press, 1987), 17–48.
22 Numbers, 93; Richard H. Shryock, "Sylvester Graham and the Popular Health Movement," *Mississippi Valley Historical Review* 18 (Sept. 1931), 174–80; Catherine E. Beecher, *A Treatise on Domestic Economy for the Use of Young Ladies at Home* (Boston, 1841), 102–3.
23 For studies of health reform see Harvey Green, *Fit for America: Health, Fitness, Sport and American Society* (New York: Pantheon Books, 1986); James C. Whorton, *Crusaders for Fitness: The History of Health Reformers* (Princeton: Princeton University Press, 1982); and John C. Burnham, "Change in the Popularization of Health in the United States," *Bulletin of the History of Medicine* 58 (Summer, 1984), 183–97.
24 Bushman and Bushman, 1233–36, Beecher quotation on p. 1218.
25 Ibid., 1228.
26 John H. Griscom, *The Sanitary Condition of the Laboring Population of New York with Suggestions for Its Improvement* (New York: Arno Press, 1970, reprint of 1845 edition), 7; Barbara Gutmann Rosenkrantz, *Public Health and the State: Changing Views in Massachusetts, 1842–1936* (Cambridge, Mass.: Harvard University Press, 1972), 29–34.
27 Charles E. Rosenberg, *The Cholera Years: The United States in 1832, 1849 and 1866* (Chicago: University of Chicago Press, 1962), 115; American Medical

Association, *First Report of the Committee on Public Hygiene* (Philadelphia: T. K. and P. G. Collins, 1849), 479–80, 568.

28 American Medical Association, 647, 479, 569; Boyer, 89.

29 Joseph Lee, *Constructive and Preventive Philanthrophy* (New York: Macmillan, 1902), 182.

30 Albert W. Ely, "On the Revival of the Roman Thermae, or Ancient Public Baths," *DeBow's Review* 2 (Oct. 1846), 232, 238.

31 Bayrd Still, *Urban America: A History with Documents* (Boston: Little, Brown, 1974), 175–82; Roy Lubove, "The New York Association for Improving the Condition of the Poor: The Formative Years," *New-York Historical Society Quarterly* 43 (July 1959), 308; Boyer, 88–93.

32 Lubove, 308; Mayor's Committee of New York City, *Report on Public Baths and Comfort Stations* (New York, 1897), 26–27; "The Benevolent Institutions of New York," *Putnam's Monthly* (June, 1853), 679; Robert Ernst, *Immigrant Life in New York, 1825–1863* (Port Washington, N.Y.: Ira J. Friedman, Inc., 1965), 51.

33 New York Association for Improving the Condition of the Poor (hereafter AICP), *Sixteenth Annual Report* (New York: John F. Trow, 1859), 57; *Twenty-fifth Annual Report* (New York, Trow and Smith, 1868), 33–34; Ernst, 51.

34 Green, 106–7.

35 Boyer, 123–25; U.S. Bureau of the Census, *Abstract of the Twelfth Census of the United States,* 3d edition (Washington, D.C.: Government Printing Office, 1904), 104; Morton Keller, *Affairs of State: Public Life in Late Nineteenth Century America* (Cambridge: Harvard University Press, 1977), 500.

36 City of Boston, *Report on Free Bathing Facilities* (City Document No. 102, 1866), 2–14.

37 Ibid.; Jane A. Stewart, "Boston's Experience with Municipal Baths," *American Journal of Sociology* 7 (Nov. 1901), 417.

38 Mayor's Committee of New York City, 27–30; T. M. B. Cross, "Report on Existing Baths in New York," supplement no. 6, Tenement House Committee of 1894, *Report* (Albany: James B. Lyon, 1895), 188; *Evening Post* (New York), May 1, 1914.

39 *Evening Post* (New York), July 14, 1893, May 1, 1914; *New York Daily Tribune,* June 6, 1880, June 24, 1888.

40 William D. P. Bliss, ed., *New Encyclopedia of Social Reform* (New York: Funk and Wagnalls, 1907), 100; Franklin B. Kirkbride, "Private Initiative in Furnishing Public Bath Facilities," *Annals of the American Academy of Political and Social Science* 13 (Mar. 1899), 281.

41 *New York Daily Tribune,* Dec. 15, 1879, July 19, 1883.

42 Tenement House Committee recommendation, quoted in Mayor's Committee of New York City, 17.

## Chapter 2

1  For a discussion of the distinction between social and structural reformers, see Melvin B. Holli, *Reform in Detroit: Hazen S. Pingree and Urban Politics* (New York: Oxford University Press, 1969), 161–81; and Arthur Mann, *Yankee Reformers in the Urban Age* (Cambridge: Belknap Press of Harvard University, 1954), 3–4.

2  Paul Boyer, *Urban Masses and Moral Order in America 1820–1920* (Cambridge: Harvard University Press, 1978), 175–90; Don S. Kirschner, "The Ambiguous Legacy: Social Justice and Social Control in the Progressive Era," *Historical Reflections* 2 (Summer, 1975), 69–88; Gordon Atkins, *Health, Housing and Poverty in New York City, 1865–1898* (lithographed Ph.D. dissertation, Ann Arbor, Mich.: Edwards Brothers, 1947), 296; Robert H. Bremner, *From the Depths: The Discovery of Poverty in the United States* (New York: New York University Press, 1956), 70–71, 134, 138; Roy Lubove, *The Progressives and the Slums: Tenement House Reform in New York City, 1890–1917* (Pittsburgh: University of Pittsburgh Press, 1962), 10–11; quotations from Melvin G. Holli, "Urban Reform in the Progressive Era," in Lewis L. Gould, ed., *The Progressive Era* (Syracuse: Syracuse University Press, 1974), 141; and Arthur S. Link and Richard L. McCormick, *Progressivism* (Arlington Heights, Ill.: Harlan Davidson, 1983), 84.

3  Bremner, *From the Depths,* 62–85, 123–31.

4  Tenement House Committee of 1894, *Report* (Albany: James B. Lyon, 1895), 1–2, 47; Simon Baruch, *A Plea for Public Baths, together with an Inexpensive Method for their Hygienic Utilization,* reprint from the *Dietetic Gazette* (May 1891), 19; inspector quoted in Lubove, *Progressives and the Slums,* 25.

5  Howard D. Kramer, "The Germ Theory and the Early Public Health Program in the United Staes," *Bulletin of the History of Medicine* 22 (May-June 1948), 240–46; James H. Cassedy, "The Flamboyant Colonel Waring: An Anticontagionist Holds the American Stage in the Age of Pasteur and Koch," in Judith Walzer Leavitt and Ronald L. Numbers, eds., *Sickness and Health in America: Readings in the History of Medicine and Public Health* (Madison: University of Wisconsin Press, 1978), 305, 309–10.

6  Simon Baruch, *Plea for Public Baths,* 18–19; Moreau Morris, "More About the Public Rain-baths," *The Sanitarian* 37 (July 1896), 11; Tenement House Committee of 1894, 49; Charles Zueblin, *American Municipal Progress,* rev. ed. (New York: Macmillan, 1916), 307.

7  G. W. W. Hanger, "Public Baths in the United States," in U.S. Department of Commerce and Labor, *Bulletin of the Bureau of Labor* 9 (Washington, D.C.: Government Printing Office, 1904), 1245, 1252; Josiah Quincy, "Gymnasiums and Playgrounds," *The Sanitarian* 41 (Oct. 1898), 309; John Paton, *Public Baths* (1893), 6.

8   William Tolman, "Public Baths, or The Gospel of Cleanliness," *Yale Review*
    6 (May 1897), 51; Baruch, "Plea for Public Baths," 8, 12.

9   *Brooklyn Daily Eagle,* Apr. 8, 1902, Jan. 28, 1895; "Americanization by Bath,"
    *Literary Digest* 47 (Aug. 13, 1913), 281; Free Bath and Sanitary League, *Round-
    up for 1897 on the Free Public Baths of Chicago* (Chicago, 1897), 16.

10  Moses Rischin, *The Promised City: New York's Jews 1870–1914* (New York:
    Harper and Row, 1970), 87; David Ward, *Cities and Immigrants* (New York:
    Oxford University Press, 1971), 109–10.

11  Lawrence Veiller, *Housing Reform: A Handbook for Practical Use in American
    Cities* (New York: Charities Publication Committee, 1910), 111; *New York
    Times,* July 13, 1895.

12  Quoted in Bertha H. Smith, "The Public Bath," *The Outlook* 79 (Mar. 4,
    1905), 576–77; *Philadelphia North American,* July 5, 1902.

13  *Rochester Herald,* quoted in *Brooklyn Daily Eagle,* Sept. 12, 1897; *New York
    Daily Tribune,* Feb. 7, 1897; Free Public Bath Commission of Baltimore,
    Maryland, *Annual Report, 1903* (Baltimore, 1904), 10.

14  Tenement House Committee of 1894, 50; Mayor's Committee of New York
    City, *Report on Public Baths and Public Comfort Stations* (New York, 1897), 9;
    *Baltimore Sun,* Dec. 7, 1898.

15  Public Baths Association of Philadelphia, *Annual Report, 1898,* 9; *Baltimore
    Sun,* Aug. 1, 1909; Free Public Baths Commission of Baltimore, Maryland,
    *Annual Report, 1913* (Baltimore, 1914), 14.

16  William Paul Gerhard, *On Bathing and Different Forms of Baths* (New York:
    William T. Comstock, 1895), 16–17.

17  Edward Mussey Hartwell, "Public Baths in Europe," in Charles H. Verrill,
    ed., *Monographs on Social Economics* (Washington, D.C.: U.S. Department of
    Labor Exhibit, Pan-American Exposition, 1901), 25–26.

18  Hartwell; Hanger.

19  Tenement House Committee of 1894, 47; Robert Coit Chapin, *The Standard
    of Living Among Workingmen's Families in New York City* (New York: William F.
    Fell, 1909), 79.

20  Jacob A. Riis, *The Battle with the Slum* (New York: Macmillan, 1902), 103,
    144; Lubove, 123.

21  *Brooklyn Daily Eagle,* Aug. 12, 1900; Smith, 568–69; M. N. Baker, *Municipal
    Engineering and Sanitation* (New York, Macmillan, 1906), 211.

22  Blake McKelvey, *The Urbanization of America, 1860–1915* (New Brunswick,
    N.J.: Rutgers University Press, 1963), 150; William H. Tolman and William
    I. Hull, *Handbook of Sociological Information with Especial Reference to New York
    City* (New York, G. P. Putnam's Sons, 1894), 254–57; Rischin, 208.

23  Tenement House Committee of 1894, 190–91; New York Association for
    Improving the Condition of the Poor, *The People's Baths* (n.d.), 5–7; idem, *The*

*People's Baths: A Study on Public Baths* (reprint from *AICP Notes,* No. 2), 2–11; *Evening Post* (New York), July 8, 1899; *New York Daily Tribune,* Aug. 18, 1891; *Boston Herald,* June 10, 1896; T. M. B. Cross, "Report on Existing Baths in New York," supplement no. 6, Tenement House Committee of 1894, 193–99. "Cleanliness is, indeed, next to Godliness" appeared in John Wesley's Sermon 93, "On Dress" and really applies to apparel rather than to the body. The entire quotation is "Let it be observed, that slovenliness is no part of religion; that neither this nor any text of Scripture condemns neatness of apparel. Certainly this is a duty, not a sin. Cleanliness is, indeed, next to godliness." John Bartlett, *Familiar Quotations,* Emily Morison Beck, ed., (Boston, Little, Brown, 1980), 346; poem published in *Tribune,* Aug. 18, 1891. For the People's Baths, see also Community Service Society Papers, box 21, folder 45. The AICP closed the People's Baths on Jan. 5, 1909, due to declining attendance and the opening of municipal baths on the Lower East Side: Community Service Society Papers, box 74, Minutes of the Committee on Public Baths, Dec. 15, 1908, and AICP, *Sixty-sixth Annual Report* (New York, 1909), 75.

24   *Brooklyn Daily Eagle,* July 2, 1893; Wiliam H. Tolman, *Social Engineering* (New York: McGraw, 1909), 62.

25   William Paul Gerhard, *The Modern Rain Bath* (New York: S. J. Parkhill, 1894), 1–3.

26   Hartwell, 32–36, quotation on p. 17; *New York Times,* July 13, 1895; M. N. Baker, *Municipal Engineering,* 210; *New York Daily Tribune,* Feb. 24, 1896.

27   Quincy quotation in City of Boston, Statistics Department, *City Record* (Oct. 20, 1898), 1:593; Christopher Tunnard and Henry Hope Reed, *American Skyline* (New York: New American Library of World Literature, 1956), 136–53; Jon A. Peterson, "The City Beautiful Movement: Forgotten Origins and Lost Meanings," *Journal of Urban History* 2 (Aug. 1976), 415–34; Boyer, 262–66; quotation on p. 264.

28   William Paul Gerhard, *The Progress of the Public Bath Movement in the United States,* paper read at the First International Conference on Public and School Baths at Scheveningen, Holland, Aug. 1912 and reprinted from *Metal Worker, Plumber and Steam Fitter,* Dec. 12, 19, 1913, 11; Hanger, 1270; Robert E. Todd, "Four New City Baths and Gymnasiums," *The Survey* 23 (Feb. 5, 1910), 680.

29   Hanger, 1266; for texts of New York State Laws, see appendixes II and III.

30   Quoted in Mayor's Committee of New York City, 59; *Evening Post* (New York), Feb. 21, 1901; Free Public Bath Commission of Baltimore, Maryland, *Annual Report, 1911* (Baltimore, 1912), 10.

31   "A New Public Bathhouse," *Charities Review* 8 (Nov. 1898), 391; Free Bath and Sanitary League, *Round-up for 1897 on the Free Public Baths of Chicago* (Chicago, 1897), 25; *New York Daily Tribune,* Aug. 7, 15, 1902.

32 See, e.g., Mayor's Committee of New York City, *Report,* 147–48; Free Public Bath Commission of Baltimore, Maryland, *Annual Report, 1905* (Baltimore, 1906), 11.

33 Zueblin, 308; John B. Walker, "Public Baths for the Poor," *Cosmopolitan* 9 (Aug. 1890), 414–18, 422.

34 Hanger, 1254–56.

35 Ibid.; Jane A. Stewart, "Model Public Bath at Brookline," *American Journal of Sociology* 5 (Jan. 1900), 470; Joseph Lee, "Municipal Baths," *Charities* 6 (Mar. 2, 1901), 184.

36 Hanger, 1254–56, 1323, 1337; B. F. Tillinghast, *Free Public Baths for Davenport* (Davenport, Iowa: Contemporary Club, 1901), 18–19.

37 Hanger, 1254–56; Civic Club of Allegheny County, *Report of Board of Managers of Bath House* (Pittsburgh, 1899), 5–6; Franklin B. Kirkbride, "Private Initiative in Furnishing Public Bath Facilities," *Annals of the American Academy of Political and Social Science* 13 (Mar. 1899), 282; Gerhard, *Progress,* 9.

38 Hanger; U.S. Census Office, *12th Census of the United States: 1900 Population,* 1:lxix; August P. Windolph, "Statistical Report on Public Baths, Laundries or Wash-houses and Comfort Stations for Municipalities of 25,000 and over in the United States," *Journal of the American Association for Promoting Hygiene and Public Baths* 4 (1922), 112–15; Gerhard, *Progress,* 38. It cannot be determined exactly how many and which cities had public baths. Windolph's article depended upon cities' response to his inquiry, and some which had baths did not respond. The AICP reported in 1912 that 40 cities had baths, although some of these may not have been open year-round. These two sources appear to show that the following cities had year-round public baths: Albany, N.Y., Baltimore, Boston, Bridgeport, Conn., Brookline, Mass., Buffalo, Cambridge, Chicago, Cleveland, Dallas, Denver, Des Moines, Detroit, Hartford, Hoboken, N.J., Holyoke, Mass., Jersey City, Kansas City, Louisville, Ky., Milwaukee, Minneapolis, Mobile, Ala., Nashville, Newark, N.J., New Bedford, Mass., Newton, Mass., New York City, Omaha, Philadelphia, Pittsburgh, Portland, Maine, Providence, R.I., Rochester, N.Y., St. Louis, St. Paul, Salt Lake City, San Francisco, Springfield, Mass., Syracuse, Taunton, Mass., Troy, N.Y., Utica, N.Y., Washington, D.C., Wilmington, Del., Worcester, Mass., Yonkers, N.Y. (AICP list of baths in unsigned letter, dated May 3, 1912, to Elsie Strong, Librarian, Bible House, CSS Papers, box 37, folder 218).

39 *Evening Post* (New York), Feb. 10, 1903; Gerhard, *Progress,* 16; A. C. Richardson, "Buffalo," *Annals of the American Academy of Political and Social Science* 26 (Nov. 1905), 157; Hanger, 1348–49.

40 For an excellent discussion of the civic symbolism of the public bath movement, see David Glassberg, "The Design of Reform: The Public Bath Move-

ment in America," *American Studies* 20 (Fall 1979), 5–21. Although incorrect in some factual details, Glassberg perceptively points out that the bath reformers wished "to extend their baptismal rites of common citizenship to all residents of their city" (6). My thanks to Jane Allen for bringing this reference to my attention.

## Chapter 3

1 *New York Daily Tribune,* Dec. 15, 1879, July 19, 1883; Mayor's Committee of New York City, *Report on Public Baths and Comfort Stations* (New York, 1897), 17, 30.

2 Benjamin Harrow, "Simon Baruch," in Allen Johnson, ed., *Dictionary of American Biography* (New York: Charles Scribner's Sons, 1929), 2:29; Frances A. Hellebrandt, *Simon Baruch: Introduction to the Man and His Work* (Richmond, Va., 1950), 12–44; Thomas E. Keys and Frank R. Krusen, "Dr. Simon Baruch and His Fight for Free Public Baths," *Archives of Physical Medicine* 26 (Sept. 1945), 549–57.

3 "Simon Baruch, M.D.," *Journal of the American Association for Promoting Hygiene and Public Baths* 4 (1922), 10; quotation from Bertha H. Smith, "The Public Bath," *Outlook* 79 (Mar. 4, 1905), 567.

4 *New York Times,* July 19, 1912, May 23, 1900; *Brooklyn Daily Eagle,* May 19, 1900; Keys and Krusen, 7; Herman B. Baruch, M.D., *The History of the Public Rain Bath in America,* reprint from *The Sanitarian* (Oct. 1896), 1.

5 Harvey E. Fisk, *The Introduction of Public Rain Baths in America, A Historical Sketch,* reprint from *The Sanitarian* (June 1896), 1–2; G. W. W. Hanger, "Public Baths in the United States," in U.S. Department of Commerce and Labor, *Bulletin of the Bureau of Labor* 9 (Washington, D.C.: Government Printing Office, 1904), 1328.

6 Fisk, 13.

7 Ibid.; for the text of this law see appendix I.

8 "Thomas F. Gilroy," *National Cyclopedia of American Biography* (New York: James T. White and Company, 1893) 3: 260; Fisk, 14; *New York Times,* Oct. 10, 1914. Otto Kempner, a staunch bath advocate, was an anti-Tammany Democrat who had been elected to the state assembly in 1892. Born in 1858, he had emigrated as a boy from Austria-Hungary with his parents, was educated at Cooper Union, and practiced law. As a political figure he constantly opposed Tammany Hall and its boss, Richard Croker. In 1898 Kempner wrote an exposé of Croker entitled *Boss Croker's Career: A Review of the Political Activity of Bill Tweed's Pupil and Successor,* which was serialized in the *New York World.* In 1897 Kempner moved to Brooklyn and in 1902 was appointed deputy commissioner of public works for that borough and was

able to participate in the building and opening of Brooklyn's first two municipal baths in 1903. See *New York Times,* Oct. 10, 1914, and *New York Daily Tribune,* Apr. 10, 23, 1894.

9   Quoted in *New York Herald,* Mar. 14, 1893; Fisk, 14.

10   George Francis Knerr, "The Mayoral Administration of William L. Strong, New York City, 1895–1897" (Ph.D. dissertation, New York University, 1957), 19–22.

11   "Richard Watson Gilder," *National Cyclopedia* 1:312–13; Tenement House Committee of 1894, *Report* (Albany: James B. Lyon, 1895), 47, quotations on 49, 75; T. M. B. Cross, "Report on Existing Baths in New York," Supplement no. 6, in Tenement House Committee of 1894, *Report,* 189–200.

12   Mayor's Committee of New York City, 21; *New York Daily Tribune,* Mar. 28, 1895; Knerr, 27–30; David C. Hammack, *Power and Society: Greater New York at the Turn of the Century* (New York: Russell Sage Foundation, 1982), 147–51; Richard Stephen Skolnik, "The Crystallization of Reform in New York City, 1890–1917," (Ph.D. dissertation, Yale University, 1964), 163–65; Richard L. McCormick, *From Realignment to Reform: Political Change in New York State, 1893–1910* (Ithaca and London: Cornell University Press, 1981), 46–47, 106. Martin J. Scheisl, *The Politics of Efficiency: Municipal Administration and Reform in America: 1880–1920* (Berkeley and Los Angeles: University of California Press, 1977), 63–64; Gerald W. McFarland, *Mugwumps, Morals and Politics, 1884–1920* (Amherst: University of Massachusetts Press, 1975), 100, 118.

13   Knerr, 31; Mayor's Committee of New York City, 22.

14   Knerr, 35–36; Hammack, 148–49.

15   *New York Times,* Jan. 24, 1913; March 18, 1904; "William H. Tolman," *National Cyclopedia* 14:219.

16   *New York Times,* Sept. 8, 1913, June 20, 1912, Apr. 21, 1916; Hammack, 178.

17   Herman B. Baruch, 3; Faure's cryptic letter to Baruch, reprinted in this article by Baruch's son, is here quoted in its entirety:

Dear Sir:

Your letter of Nov. 26, in response to my call on you, was duly received, and while it was impossible for those charged with the formation of the various subcommittees to know exactly upon what lines they might decide to work, yet it was deemed inexpedient to hamper them in advance with any conditions, and furthermore, knowing your great research of and important labors in the subject of baths and lavatories, I did not feel at liberty to take any step that might interfere with the fruition or development of your ideas, the importance of which are so well known to the public. While for these reasons we felt ourselves unable to name you as a member of the Committee, yet I trust that when the Committee shall have organized it may not be deprived of the benefit of your presence and suggestions at some of its meetings.

Yours very truly,

J. M. Faure

For Committee on Baths and Lavatories

18  Committee of Seventy, Sub-Committee on Baths and Lavatories, *Preliminary Report* (1895), 6–7, quotation on 6. The recommended sites were (1) Washington and Carlisle streets, (2) Chatham Square, (3) Essex Market, (4) Tompkins Square, (5) 58th Street and 11th Avenue, and (6) 110th Street and Second Avenue.

19  Frank Tucker, "Public Baths," in Robert W. DeForest and Lawrence Veiller, eds., *The Tenement House Problem* (New York: Macmillan, 1903), 2:42; Goodwin Brown, "The System of Public Baths in the United States," *Current Literature* 29 (Aug. 1900), 194; *New York Herald,* Apr. 21, 1895; *Brooklyn Daily Eagle,* Apr. 22, 1895. The text of this law is located in appendix II.

20  *New York Times,* July 9, 13, Sept. 22, 1895; *New York Daily Tribune,* June 20, July 9, Sept. 14, Oct. 7, 1895.

21  Mayor's Committee of New York City, 163–68; quotation in *New York Times,* July 11, 1895.

22  *New York Times,* Aug. 28, 1895; *New York Daily Tribune,* Aug. 28, 1895.

23  Tucker, 46–47; *New York Times* May 11, 1897. The text of this law is located in appendix III.

24  Mayor's Committee of New York City, 173; *New York Daily Tribune* May 27, 28, 1896; *New York Times,* May 27, 28, 31, June 6, 1896, July 2, 1904.

25  "William H. Tolman," 219; Mayor's Committee of New York City, passim, quotations on 9 and 5; William H. Tolman, "Public Baths, or the Gospel of Cleanliness," *Yale Review* 6 (May 1897), 55. The report mainly concerned the question of public baths and devoted only 27 pages out of 249 to the question of public comfort stations, a division which frequently occurred in the municipal bath movement, as has been noted. New York's bath reformers wanted the city to build public comfort stations, but the cause of public baths occupied most of their attention and efforts.

26  *New York Daily Tribune,* Feb. 7, 1897; *New York Times,* Feb. 14, 1897.

27  *New York Times,* May 11, June 4, 5, 7, 1897; Tucker, 34; New York City, Borough of Manhattan, Public Works Department, *Statistics Relating to Public Baths and Comfort Stations under the Supervision of the President of the Borough of Manhattan* (New York: Martin B. Brown Press, 1907), 3.

28  Citizens' Union, pamphlet no. 1, *Public Baths and Lavatories* (Citizens' Union, 1897); "R. Fulton Cutting," *National Cyclopedia* 45:459; Hammack, 151; McFarland, 103–4.

29  Knerr, 284–88; Hammack, 151–54; Gerald Kurland, "The Amateur in Politics: The Citizens' Union Greater New York Mayoral Campaign of 1897," *New-York Historical Society Quarterly* 53 (Oct. 1969), 352–84.

30  Ralph D. Paine, "Bathers of the City," *Outing* 46 (Aug. 1905), 569; *New York Daily Tribune,* May 7, 14, 1899.

31  *Brooklyn Daily Eagle,* June 8, 1899; *Evening Post* (New York), July 29, 30, 1901.

32  Knerr, 284–89.

33  *New York Daily Tribune,* Dec. 21, 23, 1900; AICP quotation in Tucker, 49; *Evening Post* (New York), Feb. 15, 1901.

34  *Evening Post* (New York), Feb. 15, 1901; *New York Daily Tribune,* Dec. 22, 1900; Kearny quotation in *Evening Post* (New York), Mar. 6, 1901.

35  *New York Daily Tribune,* Apr. 7, 1901; *Evening Post* (New York), Feb. 21, Mar. 30, July 20, 22, 24, 1901.

36  *Evening Post* (New York), Aug. 1, 1901; *New York Daily Tribune,* quotation in Aug. 2, 4, 1901.

37  *Evening Post* (New York), Aug. 5, 8, Oct. 10, 1901; *New York Daily Tribune,* Aug. 7, 1901.

38  Lincoln Steffens, *The Shame of the Cities* (New York: Hill & Wang, 1957), 200; Hammack, 154–57; Steven C. Swett, "The Test of a Reformer: A Study of Seth Low," *New-York Historical Society Quarterly* 44 (Jan. 1960), 29–41.

39  New York Association for Improving the Condition of the Poor, *Communication on a System of Municipal Baths for the Borough of Manhattan, City of New York, to the Honorable Jacob A. Cantor, President of the Borough,* Feb. 25, 1902, 9, 12–22; Public Baths Association of Philadelphia, *Annual Report, 1898,* 5. The suggested sites were *Below Houston Street* (1) block of James, Oak, Roosevelt, and Madison streets, (2) block of Chrystie, Forsyth, Bayard, and Canal streets, (3) block of Delancy, Broome, Essex, and Ludlow streets, (4) block of Madison, Monroe, Clinton, and Montgomery streets, (5) block of Elizabeth, Mott, Prince, and Houston streets; *Above Houston—East Side* (1) block of avenues A and B and 2nd and 3rd streets, (2) block of avenues A and B, 15th and 16th streets, (3) 2nd Avenue and 35th and 36th streets, (4) 2nd Avenue and 48th and 49th streets, (5) 1st Avenue and 58th and 59th streets, (6) 1st and 2nd avenues and 73rd and 74th streets, (7) 1st and 2nd avenues and 110th and 111th streets; *Above Houston—West Side* (1) 31st and 32nd streets and 9th and 10th avenues, (2) 9th Avenue and 40th and 41st streets, (3) block of 9th and 10th avenues and 48th and 49th streets, (4) 10th Avenue near 59th Street.

40  *New York Daily Tribune,* Mar. 3, 1902.

41  Ibid.; "Charles Sprague-Smith," *National Cyclopedia* 34:148–49; "Public Interest in Public Baths," *Charities* 8 (April 26, 1902), 382.

42  *Brooklyn Daily Eagle,* Mar. 26, 28, Apr. 7, 1902; quotation in Apr. 8, 1902.

43  *Brooklyn Daily Eagle,* June 13, 1902; *New York Daily Tribune,* Mar. 19, 1902.

44  *New York Times,* Aug. 13, 1902; *Brooklyn Daily Eagle,* Aug. 16, quotation in
    Aug. 22, Sept. 27, 1902; Deborah Bershad, Art Commission of the City of
    New York, *New York Re-viewed: Nineteenth and Early Twentieth Century Pho-
    tographs from the Collection of the Art Commission* (New York, 1985), 13. The sites
    chosen in Brooklyn were Hicks Street in South Brooklyn and Pitkin Avenue
    in Brownsville, and in Manhattan were Allen Street in the red light district,
    East 109th Street in Little Italy, and West 41st Street in the Tenderloin
    district.

45  *Brooklyn Daily Eagle,* June 15, 28, July 18, Aug. 16, Oct. 8, 1902; *New York
    Daily Tribune,* July 27, Aug. 16, 1902; *New York Times,* Aug. 13, 1902.

46  *New York Daily Tribune,* June 22, 1902, Nov. 24, 1903; *New York Times,* Feb.
    22, 1921; Philip S. Platt, "A Model Wet-Wash Laundry," *American City* 11
    (Nov. 1914), 368–69. The Milbank Memorial Bath was closed in 1919 due to
    declining patronage, but the laundry continued to operate until 1925 (Com-
    munity Service Society Papers, box 54, folders 325-11-C and 325-11). One of
    the patrons of the Milbank bath wrote to the AICP objecting to its closing:
    "It will be missed by hundreds of working men in the neighborhood who
    depended on the bath after a hard days work. . . . Why not charge a few
    cents more and keep them {sic} open" (CSS Papers, box 48, folder 325-1a).

47  *New York Daily Tribune,* Sept. 29, Oct. 25, Nov. 24, 1903; *New York Times,*
    Mar. 20, 1974, Nov. 30, 1988, June 29, 1990.

48  Allen Nevins and John A. Kraut, eds., *The Greater City: New York 1898–1948*
    (New York: Columbia University Press, 1948), 69–71. By legislative action
    the mayoralty had been given a two-year term.

49  *New York Times,* May 21, 1904; J. Joseph Huthmacher, "Charles Evans
    Hughes and Charles Francis Murphy: the Metamorphosis of Progres-
    sivism," *New York History* 46 (Jan. 1965), 28–34; Otis A. Pease, "Urban
    Reformers in the Progressive Era: A Reassessment," *Pacific Northwest Quar-
    terly* 62 (Apr. 1971), 56–57.

50  New York City, Borough of Manhattan, Public Works Department, *Public
    Baths under the Supervision of the President of the Borough of Manhattan* (1914), 19;
    New York City, Department of Parks, *Annual Report, 1916,* 109.

51  Rischin, *Promised City,* 76–78; Federal Writers' Project, *The WPA Guide to
    New York City* (New York: Pantheon Books, 1982, orig. pub. 1939), 151, 155,
    227–28, 243, 248–49; "Reasons for Small Attendance" (Nov. 9, probably
    1907), CSS Papers, box 37, folder 218.

52  *New York Times,* Aug. 13, 1902; Federal Writers' Project, 164.

53  *Evening Post* (New York), Nov. 27, 1905.

54  Frank E. Wing, "The Popularization of a Public Bath-house," *Charities* 14
    (April 29, 1905), 694–96.

55   Robert E. Todd, "The Municipal Baths of Manhattan," *Charities* 19 (Oct. 19, 1907), 897, quotation on 899; Robert E. Todd, "Four New City Baths and Gymnasiums," *The Survey* 23 (Feb. 5, 1910), 680.

56   *Evening Post* (New York), May 1, 1913.

57   B. J. Corcoran, "Public Baths of Manhattan," *Journal of the American Association for Promoting Hygiene and Public Baths* 11 (1929), 35.

58   New York City, *Statistics,* 4; *Annual Report of the Business and Transactions of the President of the Borough of Manhattan, City of New York for the Year Ending Dec. 31, 1915,* 153; New York City, Miscellaneous file entitled "New York City Baths" in Municipal Reference Library of New York City; *Report of the Business and Transactions of the President of the Borough of Manhattan, City of New York, Henry H. Curran, President, for the Year Ending Dec. 31, 1920* (New York: M. B. Brown, 1921), 14; New York City, *Public Baths,* 16.

59   Lubove, 134; *Evening Post* (New York), Mar. 24, 1917; Lawrence Veiller, *Housing Reform: A Handbook for Practical Use in American Cities* (New York: Charities Publication Committee, 1910), 112. Veiller states that after eight years of operation of the Tenement House Law of 1901, private baths for each family were provided by builders of their own volition in 86 percent of all new apartment buildings. Letter from R. E. Taylor to William H. Allen, General Agent, Dec. 12, 1906, CSS Papers, box 37, folder 218.

60   The American Association for Promoting Hygiene and Public Baths is discussed in detail in chap. 6. C. W. Williams, "City Provides Better Baths for Manhattanites," *American City* (July 1941), 69; *New York Times,* Apr. 9, 1964, July 4, 1975.

### Chapter 4

1   *Boston Herald,* Oct. 15, 1898; Boston, *City Record* 1 (Oct. 20, 1898), 593.

2   Oscar Handlin, *Boston's Immigrants,* rev. and enlarged ed. (New York: Atheneum, 1972), 108–17; Joseph Lee, *Constructive and Preventive Philanthropy* (New York: Macmillan, 1902), 182; City of Boston, *Report on Free Bathing Facilities,* City Document no. 2 (1866), 2–14; Jane A. Stewart, "Boston's Experience with Municipal Baths," *American Journal of Sociology* 7 (Nov. 1901), 417; G. W. W. Hanger, "Public Baths in the United States," in U.S. Department of Commerce and Labor, *Bulletin of the Bureau of Labor* 9 (Washington, D.C.: Government Printing Office, 1904), 1277; for text of the Massachusetts bath law see appendix IV.

3   Allen F. Davis, *Spearheads for Reform: The Social Settlements and the Progressive Movement, 1890–1914* (New York: Oxford University Press, 1967), 174–75.

4   Arthur Mann, *Yankee Reformers in the Urban Age* (Cambridge: Belknap Press of Harvard University, 1954), 115–17.

5   Ibid., 121.

6   "Josiah Quincy," *National Cyclopedia of American Biography* (New York: James T. White, 1926), 19:435; Peter d'A. Jones, "Josiah Quincy," in Melvin G. Holli and Peter d'A. Jones, eds., *Biographical Dictionary of American Mayors, 1820–1980* (Westport, Conn.: Greenwood Press, 1981), 298; *Boston Herald,* Jan. 6, 1896.

7   Geoffrey Blodgett, *The Gentle Reformers: Massachusetts Democrats in the Cleveland Era* (Cambridge: Harvard University Press, 1966), 244–54, quotation on 253–54; and "Yankee Leadership in a Divided City: Boston, 1860–1890," *Journal of Urban History* 8 (Aug. 1982), 389.

8   A. Chester Hanford, "The Government of the City of Boston, 1880–1930," in Elisabeth M. Herlihy, ed., *Fifty Years of Boston, A Memorial Volume* (Boston: Subcommittee on Memorial History of the Boston Tercentenary Committee, 1932), 84–86; Blodgett, *Gentle Reformers,* 243.

9   *Boston Herald,* Jan. 7, 21, 1896.

10  "Edward Mussey Hartwell," *Municipal Affairs* 1 (Sept. 1897), 603.

11  Ethel M. Johnson, "Labor Progress in Boston, 1880–1930," in Herlihy, *Fifty Years,* 218–19, 223; Robert Sklar, "Mary Morton Kimball Kehew," in Janet Wilson James and Paul Boyer, eds., *Notable American Women 1607–1950* (Cambridge: Harvard University Press, 1971), 2:313–14; Boston, *City Record* 1 (Oct. 20, 1898), 595.

12  Boston, *City Record* 1 (Oct. 20, 1898), 595; Wells Memorial Association, *Annual Report, 1883* (Cambridge, Mass.: Riverside Press, 1883), 2–5.

13  Boston, *City Record,* 595; *Boston Herald,* June 9, 1896.

14  *Boston Herald,* June 9, 1896.

15  Ibid.

16  Boston, *City Record,* 595–96; *Boston Herald,* Nov. 30, 1896.

17  *Boston Herald,* June 9, 1896; Mayor's Committee of New York City, *Report on Public Baths and Comfort Stations* (New York, 1897), 59–60; City of Boston, Department of Baths (hereafter referred to as BDB), *Annual Report, 1906–7* (Boston: Municipal Printing Office, 1907), 2.

18  Josiah Quincy, "Municipal Progress in Boston," *Independent* 52 (Feb. 15, 1900), 424; *Boston Herald,* Nov. 30, 1896.

19  BDB, *Annual Report, 1899–1900* (Boston: Municipal Printing Office, 1900), 2–4, 13; Robert A. Woods and Albert J. Kennedy, *The Zone of Emergence: Observations of the Lower Middle and Upper Working Class Communities of Boston, 1905–1914,* Sam Bass Warner, Jr., ed. (Cambridge and London: MIT Press, 1969), 200.

20  *Boston Herald,* Oct. 15, 1898; Boston, *City Record,* 593–95.

21  Stewart, "Boston's Experience," 418; BDB, *Annual Report, 1901–2,* 10; idem, *Annual Report, 1904–1905,* 5.

22  Josiah Quincy, "Playgrounds, Baths and Gymnasia," *Journal of Social Science* 36 (Dec. 1898), 139–40; BDB, *Annual Report, 1902–3,* 3; Blodgett, *Gentle Reformers,* 259; Lawrence Veiller, *Housing Reform: A Handbook for Practical Use in American Cities* (New York: Charities Publication Committee, 1910), 111–12.

23  Blodgett, *Gentle Reformers,* 258–59; idem, "Yankee Leadership," 389; Martin J. Schiesl, *The Politics of Efficiency: Municipal Administration and Reform in America 1880–1920* (Berkeley: University of California Press, 1977), 70; John Koren, *Boston, 1822–1922: The Story of Its Government and Principal Activities During One Hundred Years* (Boston: City of Boston Printing Department, 1923), 55.

24  Robert V. Sparks, "Thomas N. Hart," in Holli and Jones, *Biographical Dictionary,* 152; Peter d'A. Jones, "Patrick Andrew Collins," in ibid., 74.

25  BDB, *Annual Report, 1901–2,* 60; BDB, *Annual Report, 1901–3,* 5; BDB, *Annual Report, 1905–6,* 1.

26  Peter d'A. Jones, "John F. Fitzgerald," in Holli and Jones, *Biographical Dictionary,* 117; BDB, *Annual Report, 1907–8,* 4–5; BDB, *Annual Report, 1902–3,* 3; Koren, 62; William M. DeMarco, *Ethnics and Enclaves: Boston's Italian North End* (Ann Arbor, Mich.: UMI Research Press, 1980), 22–23.

27  Jones, "John F. Fitzgerald," 117; John Henry Cutler, *"Honey Fitz": Three Steps to the White House: The Colorful Life and Times of John F. ("Honey Fitz") Fitzgerald* (Indianapolis and New York: Bobbs-Merrill Company, 1962), 149–50.

28  Delos F. Wilcox, *Great Cities in America* (New York: Macmillan, 1910), 381; Koren, 59; Boston Finance Commission, *Final Report* (Boston: Committee of One Hundred, 1909), 1; Constance K. Burns, "The Irony of Progressive Reform: Boston 1898–1910," in Ronald P. Formisano and Constance K. Burns, eds., *Boston 1700–1980: The Evolution of Urban Politics,* (Westport, Conn.: Greenwood Press, 1984), 149–50; Schiesl, *Politics of Efficiency,* 102–4; Peter d'A. Jones, "George Albee Hibbard," in Holli and Jones, *Biographical Dictionary,* 162.

29  Wilcox, 388–91; Koren, 60; Jones, "George Albee Hibbard," 162; idem, "James Michael Curley," in ibid., 87; Schiesl, 104–6.

30  Charles H. Trout, "Curley of Boston: The Search for Irish Legitimacy," in Formisano and Burns, 178–81; Jones, "Curley," 87; Boston, Park and Recreation Department, *Annual Report for the Year Ending January 31, 1916,* 31–32, 46.

31  Pauline Chase Harrell and Margaret Supplee, *Victorian Boston Today* (Boston: New England Chapter, Victorian Society of America, 1975), 13–17, 25; Woods and Kennedy, *Zone of Emergence,* 147–61, 170–86; Thomas H. O'Connor, *South Boston, My Home Town: The History of an Ethnic Neighborhood* (Boston: Quinlan Press, 1988), 70–71, 86–87; Mary Antin, *The Promised Land* (Boston: Houghton Mifflin, 1912), 287, 339.

32  Woods and Kennedy, 120–44 passim (quotation on p. 143), 189–205 passim, 212; John Daniels, *In Freedom's Birthplace* (New York: Arno Press and the New York Times, 1969, orig. pub. 1914), 145–47; DeMarco, *Ethnics and Enclaves*, 15–16, 22–23.

33  BDB, *Annual Report, 1908–9*, 3–4; Hanford, "Government," 109.

34  Boston, Statistics Department, *Monthly Bulletin* (Dec. 1901), n.p.; Boston, Park and Recreation Department, *Annual Report for the Year Ending January 31, 1915*, 51, and *Annual Report for the Year Ending January 31, 1920*, 94; BDB, *Annual Report, 1899–1900*, 8; BDB, *Annual Report, 1906–7*, 14–15; BDB, *Annual Report, 1908–9*, 5; Boston Finance Commission, 32. For example in 1906–7 the superintendent of baths was provided with an automobile which cost $1,275, a chauffeur who was paid $435, plus $737 for auto repairs.

35  Jon C. Teaford, *The Unheralded Triumph: City Government in America, 1870–1900* (Baltimore and London: Johns Hopkins University Press, 1984), 311–12; Blodgett, *Gentle Reformers*, 282; Richard M. Abrams, *Conservatives in a Progressive Era: Massachusetts Politics 1900–1912* (Cambridge: Harvard University Press, 1964), 2–3; Wilcox, 372; George C. Hooker, "Mayor Quincy of Boston," *Review of Reviews* 19 (May 1899), 576–78; *Baltimore Sun*, Dec. 7, 1898. My thanks to Jack Tager for stressing, in his comments on an earlier version of this chapter, the importance of social reforms in the administrations of Fitzgerald and Curley.

36  Louis Antonellis, Parks and Recreation Department, Boston, Mass., letter, Nov. 5, 1971, to the author.

37  Free Bath and Sanitary League, *Round-up for 1897 on the Free Public Baths of Chicago* (Chicago, 1897), 13.

38  The literature on women and reform in the Progressive Era is extensive. See Judith Papachristou, *Bibliography in the History of Women in the Progressive Era* (Bronxville, N.Y.: Sarah Lawrence College Women's Studies Publication, 1985), 24–31; for women and municipal reform see Mary Ritter Beard, *Women's Work in Municipalities* (New York and London: D. Appleton, 1915); Jill Conway, "Women Reformers and American Culture, 1870–1930," *Journal of Social History* 5 (Winter 1971–72), 164–77; Paula Baker, "The Domestication of Politics: Women and American Political Society, 1780–1920," *American Historical Review* 89 (June 1984), 640–41; Carroll Smith-Rosenberg, *Disorderly Conduct: Visions of Gender in Victorian America* (New York and Oxford: Oxford University Press, 1985), 173–75; Marilyn Gitell and Teresa Shtob, "Changing Women's Roles in Political Volunteerism and Reform of the City," *Signs* 5 (Spring 1980), 569–71; and Sheila M. Rothman, *Women's Proper Place: A History of Changing Ideals and Practices, 1870 to the Present* (New York: Basic Books, 1978), 106–27; on women's clubs and urban reform see

Karen J. Blair, *The Clubwoman as Feminist: True Womanhood Redefined, 1868–1914* (New York: Holmes and Meier, 1980), 73–119; Theodora Penny Martin, *The Sound of Our Own Voices: Women's Study Clubs, 1860–1910* (Boston: Beacon Press, 1987), 173–77; Margaret Gibbons Wilson, *The American Woman in Transition: The Urban Influence, 1870–1920* (Westport, Conn.: Greenwood Press, 1979) 95–105; and Kenneth L. Kusmer, "The Functions of Organized Charity in the Progressive Era: Chicago as a Case Study," *Journal of American History* 60 (Dec. 1973), 657–78.

39   Frances Willard, letter quoted in Aileen Kraditor, *The Ideas of the Woman Suffrage Movement 1890–1920* (Garden City, N.Y.: Anchor-Doubleday, 1971), fn. 34, p. 63; Jane Addams, "Why Women Should Vote," *Ladies Home Journal* (Jan. 1910), 21; idem, *A Centennial Reader,* ed. Emily Cooper Johnson (New York, Macmillan, 1960), 114; for discussions of municipal housekeeping see Beard, *Women's Work;* Marlene Stein Wortman, "Domesticating the Nineteenth Century City," *Prospects: An Annal of American Cultural Studies* 3 (1977), 531–72; and Suellen M. Hoy, "Municipal Housekeeping: The Role of Women in Improving Urban Sanitation Practices 1800–1917," in Martin V. Melosi, ed., *Pollution and Reform in American Cities, 1870–1930* (Austin and London: University of Texas Press, 1980), 173–98.

40   Quotation from Chicago, Department of Health, *Biennial Report, 1904–1905* (Chicago, 1906), 217.

41   William H. Tolman, *Municipal Reform Movements in the United States* (New York, Fleming H. Revell, 1895), 122; Free Bath and Sanitary League, *Round-up for 1897,* 15–16; Lucy Cleveland, "The Public Baths of Chicago," *Modern Sanitation* 5 (Oct. 1908), 5–6; Carroll D. Wright, *The Slums of Baltimore, Chicago, New York and Philadelphia,* Seventh Special Report of the Commissioner of Labor (Washington, D.C.: Government Printing Office, 1894), 94.

42   Thomas Neville Bonner, "Sarah Hackett Stevenson," in *Notable American Women,* 3:374–76; Kathleen D. McCarthy, *Noblesse Oblige: Charity and Cultural Philanthropy in Chicago, 1849–1929* (Chicago and London: University of Chicago Press, 1982), 46–47; *New York Times,* Aug. 15, 1909.

43   *Medical and Surgical Register of the United States and Canada* (Detroit and Chicago: R. L. Polk, 1898), 138, 447; Paul Starr, *The Social Transformation of American Medicine* (New York: Basic Books, 1982), 99–102; Martin Kaufman, *Homeopathy in America: The Rise and Fall of a Medical Heresy* (Baltimore and London: Johns Hopkins University Press, 1971), 156–73. No information can be located on Wellington's medical practice.

44   Regina Markell Morantz, "'The Connecting Link': The Case for the Woman Doctor in 19th Century America," in Judith Walzer Leavitt and Ronald L. Numbers, eds., *Sickness and Health in America: Readings in the His-*

*tory of Medicine and Public Health* (Madison: University of Wisconsin Press, 1978), 121–23, first quotation on p. 123; Regina Markell Morantz-Sanchez, *Sympathy and Science: Women Physicians in American Medicine* (New York: Oxford University Press, 1985), 282–312, second quotation on p. 282; Mary Roth Walsh, *Doctors Wanted: No Women Need Apply: Sexual Barriers in the Medical Profession, 1835–1975* (New Haven: Yale University Press, 1977), 259–60.

45  Hanger, *Public Baths,* 1313; Cleveland, "Baths of Chicago," 7–8, quotations on p. 7; Jane Addams, *Twenty Years at Hull House* (New York: Macmillan, 1937), 313; Free Bath and Sanitary League, *Round-up,* 14–16.

46  *Chicago Tribune,* Jan. 10, 1894.

47  "Martin B. Madden," *National Cyclopedia of American Biography* (New York: James T. White, 1948), 34:420.

48  Harvey E. Fisk, *The Introduction of Public Rain Baths in America: A Historical Sketch,* reprint from *The Sanitarian,* June 1896, 7; *The Inter Ocean,* Feb. 1, 1893; *Chicago Evening Post,* Feb. 22, 1893; *The Journal,* Feb. 22, 1893; *Chicago Tribune,* Feb. 23, 1893; *The Herald,* Feb. 26, 1893.

49  Wilcox, *Great Cities,* 188, 194, quotation on p. 201; Lincoln Steffens, *The Shame of the Cities* (New York: Hill & Wang, 1957), 162–94, quotation on p. 162; Lloyde Wendt and Herman Kogan, *Bosses in Chicago: The Story of Bathhouse John and Hinky Dink* (Bloomington: Indiana University Press, 1967), 16–18.

50  Bessie Louise Pierce, *A History of Chicago* (New York: Alfred A. Knopf, 1957), 3:376–77; The Inter Ocean, *A History of Chicago, Its Men and Institutions* (Chicago: The Inter Ocean, 1900), 24–26; Edward H. Mazur, "Hempstead Washburne," "Carter H. Harrison," in Holli and Jones, *Biographical Dictionary,* 382, 151.

51  Edward H. Mazur, "John Patrick Hopkins," "George Bell Swift," and Andrew K. Prinz, "Carter Henry Harrison II," in Holli and Jones, 169, 352, 152; Edward R. Kantowicz, "Carter H. Harrison II: The Politics of Balance," in Paul M. Green and Melvin G. Holli, eds., *The Mayors: The Chicago Political Tradition* (Carbondale and Edwardsville: Southern Illinois University Press, 1987), 21.

52  Fisk, 7–9, quotation on p. 8; Chicago, Department of Health, *Biennial Report, 1897–98* (Chicago, 1899), 89–90.

53  *Chicago Tribune,* Jan. 10, 1894; Fisk, 9.

54  Hanger, 1313; Chicago, Department of Health, *Biennial Report, 1904–5* (Chicago, 1906), 218; Free Bath and Sanitary League, 24–25.

55  Fisk, 9; Hanger, 1314.

56  Fisk, 9–10; Hanger, 1315; Free Bath and Sanitary League, 10–11; J. David Hoeveler, Jr., "Lucy Louisa Coues Flower," in *Notable American Women* 1:635–36.

57  Henriette G. Frank and Amalie Jerome, *Annals of the Chicago Women's Club,*

*1876–1916* (Chicago: Chicago Women's Club, 1916), 5; Muriel Beadle, *The Fortnightly of Chicago: The City and Its Women 1873–1973* (Chicago: Henry Regnery, 1973), 25, 62, 316, 321; for the importance of women's networks in reform see Kathryn Kish Sklar, "Hull House in the 1890's: A Community of Women Reformers," *Signs* 10 (Summer 1985), 658–77; Estelle Freedman, "Separatism as Strategy: Female Institution Building and American Feminism 1870–1930," *Feminist Studies* 5 (Fall 1979), 512–29; and Blanche Wiesen Cook, "Female Support Networks and Political Activism: Lillian Wald, Crystal Eastman, Emma Goldman," in Linda K. Kerber and Jane DeHart-Matthews, eds., *Women's America,* 2nd ed. (New York and Oxford: Oxford University Press, 1987), 273–94.

58  Free Bath and Sanitary League, 43–46.

59  Hanger, 1315; Howard E. Wilson, *Mary McDowell: Neighbor* (Chicago: University of Chicago Press, 1928), 49–50.

60  Hanger, 1315; Free Bath and Sanitary League, 34–38, quotation on p. 36.

61  Hanger, 1314.

62  Chicago, Department of Health, *Report and Handbook 1911–1918* (Chicago, 1919), 1072–74; Hanger, 1317; E. R. Pritchard, "Chicago's Free Public Baths," in Department of Health of the City of Chicago, *Biennial Report 1904–1905* (Chicago, 1906), 220.

63  Agnes Sinclair Holbrook, "Map Notes and Comments," Josefa Humpal Zeman, "The Bohemian People in Chicago," and Charles Zeublin, "The Chicago Ghetto," in *Hull House Maps and Papers* (New York: Arno Press, 1970, orig. pub. 1895), 17, 93, 115; Harvey Warren Zorbaugh, *The Gold Coast and the Slum* (Chicago: University of Chicago Press, 1929), 160–61; City of Chicago, *Historic City; the Settlement of Chicago* (Chicago: Department of Development and Planning, 1976), map titled Community Settlement 1900, n.p.

64  Allen H. Spear, *Black Chicago: The Making of a Negro Ghetto, 1890–1920* (Chicago and London: University of Chicago Press, 1967), 11–12.

65  Chicago, Department of Health, *Biennial Report 1897–98,* 89–92; *Report and Handbook, 1911–18,* 1074; *Report, 1907–1910* (Chicago, 1911), 217.

66  Chicago, Department of Health, *Report, 1907–1910,* 219, quotation on p. 216.

67  Chicago, Department of Health, *Report, 1907–1910,* 217; *Report and Handbook, 1911–1918,* 1068, 1070; *Report, 1919–21* (Chicago, 1923), 196–97; Edith Abbott, *The Tenements of Chicago, 1908–1935* (Chicago: University of Chicago Press, 1936), 61.

68  *Chicago Tribune,* Apr. 5, 1973; Robert Willoughby, Chicago Park District, letter, Aug. 22, 1989, to author.

Chapter 5

1  U.S. Census Office, *Twelfth Census of the United States: 1900 Population* (Washington, D.C.: Government Printing Office, 1903), 1:lxix.

2  Carroll D. Wright, *The Slums of Baltimore, Chicago, New York and Philadelphia,* Seventh Special Report of the Commissioner of Labor (Washington, D.C.: Government Printing Office, 1894), 94; Franklin B. Kirkbride, "Private Initiative in Furnishing Public Bath Facilities," *Annals of the American Academy of Political and Social Science* 13 (March 1899), 281; Public Baths Association of Philadelphia (hereafter referred to as PBA), *Fifth Annual Report, 1902,* 5.

3  U.S. Census Office, *Twelfth Census,* lxix.

4  Lincoln Steffens, *The Shame of the Cities* (New York, Hill and Wang, 1957), 134; Delos Wilcox, *Great Cities in America* (New York, Macmillan, 1910), 244; Philip S. Benjamin, "Gentlemen Reformers in the Quaker City, 1870–1912," *Political Science Quarterly* 85 (March 1970), 61–65.

5  Benjamin, 67–77; Nathaniel Burt and Wallace E. Davies, "The Iron Age, 1876–1905," in Russell F. Weigley, ed., *Philadelphia: A 300-Year History* (New York: W. W. Norton, 1982), 498; Lloyd M. Abernethy, "Insurgency in Philadelphia, 1905," *Pennsylvania Magazine of History and Biography* 87 (Jan. 1963), 3–20, and "Progressivism 1905–1919" in Weigley, 539–43; Donald W. Disbrow, "Reform in Philadelphia Under Mayor Blankenburg, 1912–1916," *Pennsylvania History* 27 (Oct. 1960), 379–96.

6  Wilcox, 275–76; Sam Bass Warner, Jr., *The Private City: Philadelphia in Three Periods of Its Growth* (Philadelphia: University of Pennsylvania Press, 1968), esp. p. 204; Bonnie R. Fox, "The Philadelphia Progressives: A Test of the Hofstadter Hays Theses," *Pennsylvania History* 34 (Oct. 1967), 394; Abernethy, "Progressivism," 547.

7  Kirkbride, "Private Initiative," 281; Free Public Bath Commission of Baltimore, Maryland, *Annual Report, 1912* (Baltimore: n.p., 1913), 11.

8  Wilcox, 305.

9  PBA, *Tenth Annual Report, 1907,* 5–7; Kirkbride, "Private Initiative," 282; PBA Papers, Typescript History, box 2, 72:45.

10 *People's Bath for Philadelphia, A Short Account of the Public Baths Association of Philadelphia, Its Organization and Objects, Charter and By-Laws* (Philadelphia: Times Printing House, 1895), 7–8; Kirkbride, "Private Initiative," 280.

11 *People's Baths for Philadelphia,* 28–31.

12 *New York Times,* Apr. 3, 1920; PBA, *Fifth Annual Report, 1902,* 1; New York Association for Improving the Condition of the Poor, *Communication on a System of Municipal Baths for the Borough of Manhattan, City of New York, to the Honorable Jacob A. Cantor, President of the Borough, Feb. 25, 1902;* Stanley H. Howe, *History, Condition and Needs of Public Baths in Manhattan,* NYAICP Pub-

lication No. 71, probably 1912, 4 in Community Service Society Papers, box 37, folder 218.

13  *New York Times,* Dec. 6, 1954.

14  Ibid., Sept. 29, 1955.

15  Ibid., Jan. 8, 1918; "Edward B. Smith," *National Cyclopedia of American Biography* (New York: James T. White, 1927), 17:306–7.

16  *New York Times,* Mar. 29, 1949.

17  Nathaniel Burt, *The Perennial Philadelphians: The Anatomy of an American Aristocracy* (Boston: Little, Brown, 1963), 347; Durwood Howes, ed., *American Women: The Official Who's Who Among the Women of the Nation, 1937–38* (Los Angeles: American Publications, 1937), 2:409; *New York Times,* June 24, 1957; Sarah Dickson Lowrie, *Strawberry Mansion* (Philadelphia: Committee of 1926 of Pennsylvania, 1941); PBA, Minute Book, Jan. 12, 1908, box 2, 72:45.

18  PBA, Minute Book, Feb. 27, 1923; Sidney Ratner, ed., *New Light on the History of Great American Fortunes in 1892 and 1902* (New York: Augustus M. Kelley, 1953), 49; "Charlemagne Tower," *National Cyclopedia,* 26:124–25.

19  PBA, *Annual Reports, 1898–1904, 1907, 1912, 1928–1944;* PBA, Minute Book; Ratner, 50; E. Digby Baltzell, *Philadelphia Gentlemen: The Making of a National Upper Class,* (Glencoe, Ill.: Free Press, 1958), 58, 97–98.

20  *People's Baths for Philadelphia,* 12–14; Franklin B. Kirkbride, "Philadelphia Public Baths," *Annals of the American Academy of Political and Social Science* 11 (Jan. 1898), 127; PBA, *Report for 1898,* 8–11; Maxwell Whiteman, "Philadelphia's Jewish Neighborhoods," in Allen F. Davis and Mark H. Haller, eds., *The Peoples of Philadelphia: A History of Ethnic Groups and Lower Class Life, 1790–1940* (Philadelphia: Temple University Press, 1973), 241–42; Fredric M. Miller, Morris J. Vogel, and Allen F. Davis, *Still Philadelphia: A Photographic History, 1890–1940* (Philadelphia: Temple University Press, 1983), 14–15.

21  PBA, *Report for 1898,* 7–11; *Brooklyn Daily Eagle,* July 9, 1899.

22  PBA, *Report for 1898,* 8–11; G. W. W. Hanger, "Public Baths in the United States," U.S. Department of Commerce and Labor, *Bulletin of the Bureau of Labor* 9 (Washington, D.C.: Government Printing Office, 1904), 1355; quotations from *People's Baths for Philadelphia,* 8; PBA, *Tenth Annual Report, 1907,* 9, and *15th Annual Report, 1912,* back cover.

23  Quotation from PBA, *Report for 1898,* 7; Whiteman, "Philadelphia's Jewish Neighborhoods," 242; PBA, *Tenth Annual Report, 1907,* 19.

24  PBA, *Second Annual Report, 1899,* quotation on p. 6; *Tenth Annual Report,* 19.

25  Kirkbride, "Private Initiative," 283; PBA, *Report for 1898,* 9.

26  PBA, *Third Annual Report, 1900,* 5.

27  PBA, *Fourth Annual Report, 1901,* 2–5; *Daily Evening Telegraph* (Philadelphia), Mar. 30, 1903; *Philadelphia Press,* Mar. 31, 1903.

28    W. L. Ross, "Cleanliness and Its Advertisement, the Establishment of a Wash-House for Men in Philadelphia," *Charities* 12 (April 2, 1904), 333; PBA, *Fourth Annual Report, 1901,* 5; Hanger, 1356.

29    Ross, "Cleanliness," 335; PBA, *Seventh Annual Report, 1904,* 8.

30    PBA, *Tenth Annual Report, 1907,* 19; PBA, *15th Annual Report, 1912,* 3, 5, 13–16; Miller, Vogel, and Davis, *Still Philadelphia,* 5.

31    PBA, Typescript History, 5, box 2, 72:45.

32    PBA, Minute Book, Nov. 26, 1915, Jan. 26, 1922, box 2, 72:45.

33    Ibid., Jan. 26, 1922, Mar. 26, 1924, Mar. 23, 1928.

34    Caroline Golub, "The Immigrant and the City: Poles, Italians and Jews in Philadelphia, 1870–1920," in Davis and Haller, *Peoples of Philadelphia,* 208–9; Clara A. Hardin, *The Negroes of Philadelphia: The Culture of Adjustment of a Minority Group* (Bryn Mawr, Pa.: n.p., 1945), 1; Roger Lane, *Roots of Violence in Black Philadelphia, 1860–1900* (Cambridge and London: Harvard University Press, 1986), 22.

35    PBA, *31st Annual Report, 1928,* back cover, 6; *32nd Annual Report, 1929,* back cover, 6; *33rd Annual Report, 1930,* 3; Minute Book, June 10, 1931; *34th–40th Annual Reports, 1931–1937.*

36    PBA, Minute Book, June 12, 1942; *45th Annual Report, 1942,* 3; *46th Annual Report, 1943,* 1; quotation in Minute Book, Aug. 2, 1943; Minute Book, Oct. 10, 1946, Sept. 27, 1948, Jan. 11, 1950.

37    *Proceedings of the American Association for Promoting Hygiene and Public Baths* (1916), 2; *Journal of the American Association for Promoting Hygiene and Public Baths* 4 (1922), 2; PBA, *Annual Reports.*

38    Free Public Bath Commission of Baltimore, Maryland (hereafter referred to as FPBC), *Annual Report, 1913* (Baltimore, 1914), 14.

39    James B. Crooks, *Politics and Progress: The Rise of Urban Progressivism in Baltimore 1895–1911* (Baton Rouge: Louisiana State University Press, 1968), 8–41, 226–36.

40    FPBC, *1900–1925: Twenty-fifth Anniversary of the Free Public Bath Commission of Baltimore, Maryland* (Baltimore: King Brothers, 1925), 3.

41    Ibid.; Anne Beadenkopf, "The Baltimore Public Baths and their Founder, the Rev. Thomas M. Beadenkopf," *Maryland Historical Magazine* 45 (Sept. 1950), 204–5.

42    Beadenkopf, 202–3; FPBC, *Annual Report, 1901* (Baltimore, 1901), 13; William H. Hale, "Personal Reminiscences of the Rev. Thomas M. Beadenkopf," *Proceedings of the American Association for Promoting Hygiene and Public Baths* (1916), 80.

43    Baltimore *Sun,* Aug. 3, 1928; FPBC, *Annual Report, 1900* (Baltimore, 1901), 3; Crooks, *Politics and Progress,* 229.

44    FPBC, *Twenty-fifth Anniversary,* 5; Beadenkopf, "Baltimore Public Baths," 205.

45  Crooks, *Politics and Progress*, 8–11, 26, 34, 41; Joseph L. Arnold, "Alceus Hooper," in Melvin Holli and Peter d'A. Jones, eds., *Biographical Dictionary of American Mayors, 1820–1980* (Westport, Conn.: Greenwood Press, 1981), 168.

46  Crooks, *Politics and Progress*, 8–41; "Politics and Reform: The Dimensions of Baltimore Progressivism," *Maryland Historical Magazine* 71 (Fall 1976), 421–27; Andrea R. Andrews, "The Baltimore School Building Program, 1870–1890: A Study of Urban Reform," *Maryland Historical Magazine* 70 (Fall 1975), 260–74.

47  Crooks, *Politics and Progress*, 5–7; Beadenkopf, "Baltimore Public Baths," quotation on p. 214.

48  Joseph L. Arnold, "The Neighborhood and City Hall: The Origin of Neighborhood Associations in Baltimore, 1880–1911," *Journal of Urban History* 6 (Nov. 1979), 8, 26, fn. 12.

49  Beadenkopf, "Baltimore Public Baths," 205; FPBC, *Twenty-fifth Anniversary*, 5.

50  FPBC, *Twenty-fifth Anniversary*, 5; Baltimore *Sun*, Dec. 7, 1898.

51  FPBC, *Twenty-fifth Anniversary*, 5; Baltimore *Sun*, Dec. 7, 1898.

52  FPBC, *Twenty-fifth Anniversary*, 5; Beadenkopf, "Baltimore Public Baths," 207; Crooks, *Politics and Progress*, 183.

53  FPBC, *Annual Report, 1900*, 8–9.

54  Ibid., 10–11.

55  Broadus Mitchell, "Henry Walters," in Allen Johnson, ed., *Dictionary of American Biography* (New York: Charles Scribner's Sons, 1929), 19:399.

56  FPBC, *Annual Report, 1900*, 17.

57  Ibid., 10–11.

58  Ibid., 11.

59  Ibid., 17.

60  Ibid., 13–14; Sherry H. Olson, *Baltimore: The Building of an American City* (Baltimore: Johns Hopkins University Press, 1980), 229; Baltimore *Sun*, May 19, 1900; Robert F. G. Kelley, "A Public Laundry in a Bathhouse," *American City* 26 (Jan. 1922), 44–45.

61  FPBC, *Annual Report, 1900*, 12–13; *Annual Report, 1901*, 11.

62  FPBC, *Annual Report, 1900*, 3; Crooks, *Politics and Progress*, 236; Regina Markell Morantz-Sanchez, *Sympathy and Science: Women Physicians in American Medicine* (New York: Oxford University Press, 1985), 173.

63  FPBC, *Annual Report, 1900*, 14; *Annual Report, 1901*, 7.

64  FPBC, *Annual Report, 1901*, 7; *Annual Report, 1903*, 9; *Annual Report, 1905*, 10.

65  FPBC, *Annual Report, 1901*, 13; Crooks, *Politics and Progress*, 229–36.

66  FPBC, *Annual Report, 1901*, 5–6; Baltimore *Sun*, Aug. 1, 1909.

67  FPBC, *Annual Report, 1901*, 6; *Annual Report, 1903*, 5; Beadenkopf, "Bal-

timore Public Baths," 210; Baltimoe *Sun,* Aug. 1, 1909; James B. Crooks,
"Maryland Progressivism," in Richard Walsh and William Lloyd Fox, eds.,
*Maryland: A History 1632–1974* (Baltimore: Maryland Historical Society,
1974), 661. The other exceptions were playgrounds and an African-American teachers' college.

68 FPBC, *Annual Report, 1901,* 9–10; *Twenty-fifth Anniversary,* 9; *Annual Report,
1903,* 5; *Annual Report, 1902,* 7; Baltimore *Sun,* Aug. 1, 1909.

69 FPBC, *Annual Report, 1905,* 9; *Annual Report, 1906,* 6; *Annual Report, 1909,* 7;
*Annual Report, 1914,* 8, 11; *Annual Report, 1913,* 11.

70 Kelley, "A Public Laundry," 44–45.

71 FPBC, *Annual Report, 1910,* 12–13; Olson, *Baltimore,* 279, 285–86; Baltimore
*Sun,* Apr. 13, 1911.

72 FPBC, *Annual Report, 1912,* 11; *Annual Report, 1922,* 13; *Twenty-fifth Anniversary,*
23; Olson, 229; Linda G. Rich, Joan Clark Netherwood, and Elinor B. Cahn,
*Neighborhood, a State of Mind* (Baltimore and London: Johns Hopkins University Press, 1981), 13–14.

73 FPBC, *Annual Report, 1903,* 8; *Annual Report, 1905,* 11; *Twenty-fifth Anniversary,*
21–23.

74 Beadenkopf, "Baltimore Public Baths," 212; FPBC, *Annual Report, 1906,* 5;
*Annual Report, 1907,* 10; *Annual Report, 1913,* 17; *Annual Report, 1915,* 9.

75 FPBC, *Annual Report, 1903,* 9; *Annual Report, 1908,* 7; *Annual Report, 1909,* 10;
*Annual Report, 1910,* 16; *Annual Report, 1912,* 19; *Twenty-fifth Anniversary,* 14.

76 Beadenkopf, "Baltimore Public Baths," 212–13; FPBC, *Portable Shower Baths:
A New Departure in Municipal Bath Houses,* 1–5; FPBC, *Annual Report, 1910,* 9.

77 FPBC, *Annual Report, 1905,* 11; *Annual Report, 1909,* 8; Beadenkopf, "Baltimore Public Baths," 210, 214.

78 FPBC, *Annual Reports, 1900–1928.*

79 FPBC, *Annual Report, 1912,* 11.

80 Leon Rubenstein, director, Department of Legislative Reference, Baltimore, Md., to the author, Aug. 16, 1971.

81 Robert H. Bremner, *American Philanthropy* (Chicago: University of Chicago
Press, 1960), 108–9, Carnegie quotation on p. 109; Kathleen D. McCarthy,
*Noblesse Oblige: Charity and Cultural Philanthropy in Chicago, 1849–1929* (Chi-
cago: University of Chicago Press, 1982), 152.

## Chapter 6

1 William Paul Gerhard, *The Progress of the Public Bath Movement in the United
States,* paper read at the First International Conference on Public and
School Baths at Scheveningen, Holland, Aug. 1912, reprinted from *Metal
Worker, Plumber and Steam Fitter,* Dec. 12 & 19, 1913, 1–2.

2  *Boston Herald,* Jan. 21, 1896; Lucy Cleveland, "The Public Baths of Chicago," *Modern Sanitation* 5 (Oct. 1908), 5–6; Franklin B. Kirkbride, "Philadelphia Public Baths," *Annals of the American Academy of Political and Social Science* 11 (Jan. 1898), 127; Anne Beadenkopf, "The Baltimore Public Baths and their Founder, the Rev. Thomas M. Beadenkopf," *Maryland Historical Magazine* 45 (Sept. 1950), 207.

3  See bibliography for examples.

4  Gerhard, *Progress,* 1–2; *Proceedings of the American Association for Promoting Hygiene and Public Baths* (1916), 2 (hereafter referred to as *Proceedings*); *Journal of the American Association for Promoting Hygiene and Public Baths* (hereafter referred to as *Journal*) 1 (1918), 37.

5  Proceedings, 2; *Journal* 6 (1924), 67.

6  For discussions of the professionalization of urban social reformers, see Roy Lubove, *The Professional Altruist: The Emergence of Social Work as a Career* (New York: Atheneum, 1977), and Don S. Kirschner, *The Paradox of Professionalism: Reform and Public Service in Urban America 1900–1940* (Westport, Conn.: Greenwood Press, 1986), chaps. 1 and 2.

7  *Proceedings,* 2; *Journal* 4 (1922), 15; idem, 10 (1928), 2.

8  *Journal* 6 (1924), 60; 7 (1925), 9–10; 8 (1926), 9; 10 (1928), 15.

9  Gerhard, *Progress,* 1–2; *Proceedings,* 2, 83–87; *Journal* 1 (1918); idem, 4 (1922)–11 (1929) passim.

10  Première Conférence Internationale de Bains Populaires et Scolaires tenue à Schêveningue, 27–30 Août 1912 (First International Conference on People's and School Baths, held at Scheveningen, August 27–30, 1912), *Comte-rendu de Travaux* (Amsterdam, J. H. de Bussy), xxiii; "International Conference on Public Baths," *Survey* 29 (Dec. 21, 1912), 351–52.

11  *Comte-rendu,* xii–xiii, xxv–xxxiii, 247.

12  Ibid., 18.

13  Ibid., 18, 248–49, 252; A. M. Ruysch-Douwes Dekker, "The International Association for Public Baths and Cleanliness," *Journal* 9 (1927), 6, 59; idem, 6 (1924), 11–12.

14  *Proceedings; Journal* 1 (1918); idem, 4 (1922)–11 (1929) passim.

15  *Journal* 4 (1922)–11 (1929) passim.

16  Ibid., 9 (1927), 5–6.

17  Ibid., 4 (1922), 2; 11 (1929), 2.

18  Ibid., 9 (1927), 2; 10 (1928), 3; 11 (1929), 3.

### Chapter 7

1  Civic Club of Allegheny County, *Report of the Board of Managers of the Bath House* (Pittsburgh, 1899), 9; Lily Todd Phillips, "The Branch Public Baths of

Richmond, Virginia," *Journal of the American Association for Promoting Hygiene and Public Baths* 8 (1926), 47.

2  Robert Wiebe, *Businessmen and Reform: A Study of the Progressive Movement* (Chicago: Quadrangle Books, 1968), 211–12.

3  For discussions of the issue of social control in progressive reform, see Don S. Kirschner, "The Ambiguous Legacy: Social Justice and Social Control in the Progressive Era," *Historical Reflections* 2 (Summer 1975), 69–88; Paul Boyer, *Urban Masses and Moral Order in America 1820–1920* (Cambridge: Harvard University Press, 1978), 179–90, 220–32; and Marvin E. Gettleman, "Philanthropy as Social Control in Late Nineteenth Century America: Some Hypotheses and Data on the Rise of Social Work," *Societas* 5 (Winter 1975), 49–59.

4  Josiah Quincy, "Playgrounds, Baths and Gymnasia," *Journal of Social Science* 36 (Dec. 1898), 144.

5  For a discussion of the pleasurable aspects of bathing in late nineteenth- and twentieth-century America, see Jacqueline S. Wilkie, "Submerged Sensuality: Technology and Perceptions of Bathing," *Journal of Social History* 19 (Summer 1986), 649–64.

6  In the early 1970s, when I interviewed people living at the Hebrew Home for the Aged in New York City who had lived on the Lower East Side in the early 1900s regarding their recollections of the public baths, they claimed that they had never used the public baths, which were for really poor people. Most, however, fondly remembered using the swimming pools in the public baths when they were children and adolescents.

7  For progressive attempts to control the use of leisure time by the urban poor, see Boyer, 242–51; Dominick Cavallo, *Muscles and Morals: Organized Playgrounds and Urban Reform 1880–1920* (Philadelphia: University of Pennsylvania Press, 1981); Stephen Hardy, *How Boston Played: Sport, Recreation and Community, 1865–1915* (Boston, Northeastern University Press, 1982), 99–106; and *Evening Post* (New York), Aug. 7, 1906.

8  City of Boston, Statistics Department, *City Record* 1 (Oct. 20, 1898), 593.

9  Public Baths Association of Philadelphia, *Annual Report, 1900,* 4–5; City of Boston, Department of Baths, *Annual Report, 1899–1900,* 4; *New York Daily Tribune,* June 24, 1906, 5:1.

10  Donald B. Armstrong, "Public Bath Advertising Campaign," *The Survey* 31 (Feb. 21, 1914), 646–47; Richard K. Means, *Historical Perspectives on School Health* (Thorofare, N.J.: Charles B. Stack, 1975), 30–45; Stephan E. Brumberg, *Going to America, Going to School: The Jewish Immigrant Public School Encounter in Turn-of-the-Century New York* (New York: Praeger, 1986), 76, 78. Beyond the purview of this book, but of great importance in disseminating the gospel of cleanliness, were the extensive advertising campaigns of

American manufacturers of bathroom equipment and soap. See, e.g., Richard L. Bushman and Claudia L. Bushman, "The Early History of Cleanliness in America," *Journal of American History* 74 (Mar. 1988), 1232–38, and Harvey Green, *Fit for America: Health, Fitness, Sport and American Society* (New York: Pantheon, 1986), 155–56. For the activities of the soap manufacturer's Cleanliness Institute, which were aimed at schoolchildren, see Vincent Vinikas, "Lustrum of the Cleanliness Institute, 1927–1932," *Journal of Social History* 22 (Summer 1989), 613–30.

11   For an example of the desire of the poor for bathrooms of their own, see Margaret F. Byington, *Homestead: The Households of a Mill Town* (Pittsburgh: University Center for International Studies, 1974, orig. pub. 1910), 60.

12   David Glassberg, "The Design of Reform: The Public Bath Movement in America," *American Studies* 20 (Fall 1979), 18; Wilkie, "Submerged Sensuality," 654; Lawrence Veiller, *Housing Reform: A Handbook for Practical Use in American Cities* (New York: Charities Publication Committee, 1910), 112; Siegfried Giedion, *Mechanization Takes Command* (New York: Oxford University Press, 1948), 703; Bureau of Municipal Research of Philadelphia, *Workingmen's Standard of Living in Philadelphia* (New York: Macmillan, 1919), 48, quotation on p. 47; U.S. Bureau of Labor, quoted in Leila Houghteling, *The Income and Standard of Living of Unskilled Laborers in Chicago* (Chicago: University of Chicago Press, 1927), 109.

13   Edith Abbott, *The Tenements of Chicago, 1908–1935* (Chicago: University of Chicago Press, 1936), 415; James Ford et al., *Slums and Housing* (Cambridge: Harvard University Press, 1936), 1:307–8, 2:663.

# Selected Bibliography

## Public Documents

Boston, Department of Baths. *Annual Reports, 1899–1909.* Boston: Municipal Printing Office, 1900–09.

———. *Monthly Bulletin* (Dec. 1901).

———. Park and Recreation Department. *Annual Reports for the Years Ending January 31, 1915, January 31, 1916, and January 31, 1920.* Boston: 1915, 1916, 1920.

———. *Report on Free Bathing Facilities.* City Document No. 102, 1866.

———. Statistics Department. *City Record* (Oct. 20, 1898), 1:593, 595–596.

Boston Finance Commission. *Final Report.* Boston: Committee of One Hundred, 1909.

Chicago, Department of Health. *Biennial Report, 1897–1898.* Chicago: 1899.

———. *Biennial Report for the Years 1904–1905.* Chicago, 1906.

———. *Report, 1907–1910.* Chicago, 1911.

———. *Report and Handbook, 1911–1918.* Chicago, 1919.

———. *Annual Report, 1919–1921.* Chicago, 1923.

Chicago Park District, *Annual Report, 1969.* Chicago, 1970.

Cross, T. M. B. "Report on Existing Baths in New York." Supplement No. 6, Tenement House Committee of 1894. *Report.* Albany: James B. Lyon, 1895, 188–203.

Free Public Bath Commission of Baltimore, Maryland. *Annual Reports, 1900–1928.* Baltimore, 1901–29.

———. *Portable Shower Baths: A New Departure in Municipal Bath Houses.*

———. *1900–1925: Twenty-Fifth Anniversary of the Free Public Bath Commission of Baltimore, Maryland.* Baltimore: King Brothers, 1925.

Hanger, G. W. W. "Public Baths in the United States." In U.S. Department of Commerce and Labor. *Bulletin of the Bureau of Labor,* 9, 1904. Washington: Government Printing Office, 1904, 1245–1367.

Hartwell, Edward Mussey. "Public Baths in Europe." *Monographs on Social Economics,* ed. Charles H. Verrill, No. 6. Washington, 1901. U.S. Department of Labor Exhibit, Pan-American Exposition, 1901.

Mayor's Committee of New York City. *Report on Public Baths and Public Comfort Stations.* New York, 1897.

New York City, *Annual Report of the Business and Transactions of the President of the Borough of Manhattan, City of New York for the Year Ending December 31, 1915.* New York: Clarence S. Nathan, 1916.

———. Borough of Manhattan, Public Works Department. *Public Baths Under the Supervision of the President of the Borough of Manhattan.* New York, 1914.

———. Borough of Manhattan, Public Works Department. *Statistics Relating to Public Baths and Comfort Stations Under the Supervision of the President of the Borough of Manhattan.* New York: Martin B. Brown Press, 1907.

———. Borough of Manhattan, *Report of the Business and Transactions of the President of the Borough of Manhattan, City of New York, Henry H. Curran, President, for the Year Ending Dec. 31, 1920.* New York: M. B. Brown, 1921.

———. Department of Parks. *Annual Report, 1916.*

———. Miscellaneous File entitled "New York City Baths" located in Municipal Reference Library of New York City.

Tenement House Committee of 1894. *Report.* Albany: James B. Lyon, 1895.

U.S. Bureau of the Census, *Historical Statistics of the United States, Colonial Times to 1970.* Bicentennial edition, vol. 1. Washington, D.C.: Government Printing Office, 1975.

U.S. Census Office. DeBow, J. D. B. *Statistical View of the United States: Compendium of the Seventh Census.* Washington: A. O. P. Nicholson, 1854.

U.S. Census Office. *Twelfth Census of the United States: 1900, Population,* vol. 1. Washington, D.C.: Government Printing Office, 1903.

Wright, Carroll D. *The Slums of Baltimore, Chicago, New York and Philadelphia.* Seventh Special Report of the Commissioner of Labor. Washington, D.C.: Government Printing Office, 1894.

## Newspapers

*Baltimore Sun.* 1898, 1900, 1909, 1928.

*Boston Herald.* 1896, 1898.

*Brooklyn Daily Eagle.* 1891–1902, 1949.

*Chicago Tribune.* 1894.

*Daily Evening Telegraph* (Philadelphia). 1903.

*Daily News* (New York). 1971.

*Evening Post* (New York). 1879–1921.

*New York Daily Tribune.* 1879–1906.

*New York Herald.* 1893, 1895.

*New York Times.* 1890–1920.

*Philadelphia Press.* 1903.

# Selected Bibliography

## Contemporary Sources

Addams, Jane, *Twenty Years at Hull House*. New York: Macmillan, 1937.

———. "Why Women Should Vote." *Ladies Home Journal* (Jan. 1910): 21–22.

Allsop, Robert Owen. *Public Baths and Wash-houses*. London: E. & F. N. Spon, 1894.

American Medical Association. *First Report of the Committee on Public Hygiene*. Philadelphia: T. K. and P. G. Collins, 1849.

"Americanization By Bath." *Literary Digest* 47 (Aug. 23, 1913): 280–81.

Armstrong, Donald B. "Public Bath Advertising Campaign." *The Survey* 31 (Feb. 21, 1914): 646–47.

Ashpitel, Arthur, and Whichcord, John. *Baths and Washhouses*. London: T. Richards, 1853.

Baker, M. N. *Municipal Engineering and Sanitation*. New York: Macmillan, 1906.

Baruch, Herman B., M. D. *The History of the Public Rain Bath in America*. Reprint from *The Sanitarian* (Oct. 1896).

Baruch, Simon. *A Plea for Public Baths, together with an Inexpensive Method for Their Hygienic Utilization*. Reprint from *Dietetic Gazette* (May 1891).

Beard, Mary Ritter. *Woman's Work in Municipalities*. New York and London: D. Appleton, 1915.

Beecher, Catherine E. *A Treatise on Domestic Economy for the Use of Young Ladies at Home*. Boston, 1841.

"The Benevolent Institutions of New York." *Putnam's Monthly* (June 1853): 673–86.

Bliss, William D. P., ed. *New Encyclopedia of Social Reform*. New York: Funk and Wagnalls, 1907.

Brown, Goodwin. "The System of Public Baths in the United States." *Current Literature* 29 (Aug. 1900): 194–95.

Bureau of Municipal Research of Philadelphia. *Workingmen's Standard of Living in Philadelphia*. New York: Macmillan, 1919.

Campbell, Agnes. *Report on Public Baths and Wash-houses in the United Kingdom*. Sponsored by Carnegie United Kingdom Trust. Edinburgh: T. & A. Constable, 1918.

Chapin, Robert Coit. *The Standard of Living Among Workingmen's Families in New York City*. New York: William F. Fell, 1909.

Citizens Union. *Pamphlet No. 1, Public Baths and Lavatories*. [New York:] Citizens Union, 1897.

Civic Club of Allegheny County. *Report of the Board of Managers of the Bath House*. Pittsburgh: 1899.

Cleveland, Lucy. "The Public Baths of Chicago." *Modern Sanitation* 5 (Oct. 1908): 5–17.

Committee of Seventy, Sub-committee on Baths and Lavatories. *Preliminary Report.* [New York:] 1895.

Corcoran, B. J. "Public Baths of Manhattan." *Journal of the American Association for Promoting Hygiene and Public Baths* 11 (1929): 35–41.

Cross, Alfred W. S. *Public Baths and Wash-houses.* London: B. T. Botsford, 1906.

Community Service Society Papers (includes New York Association for Improving the Condition of the Poor Papers), Rare Book and Manuscript Library, Columbia University.

Dekker, A. M. Ruysch-Dowes. "The International Association for Public Baths and Cleanliness." *Journal of the American Association for Promoting Hygiene and Public Baths* 9 (1927): 59.

Ely, Albert W. "On the Revival of the Roman Thermae, or Ancient Public Baths." *DeBows Review* 2 (Oct. 1846): 228–39.

Fisk, Harvey E. *The Introduction of Public Rain Baths in America: A Historical Sketch.* Reprint from *The Sanitarian* (June 1896).

Free Bath and Sanitary League. *Round-up for 1897 on the Free Public Baths of Chicago.* Published by Dr. Gertrude G. Wellington, president, and J. Van Allen, secretary of the league. Chicago, 1897.

Gerhard, William Paul. *Modern Baths and Bath Houses.* New York: John Wiley and Sons, 1908.

———. *The Modern Rain Bath.* New York: S. J. Parkhill, 1894.

———. *On Bathing and Different Forms of Baths.* New York: William T. Comstock, 1895.

———. "People's Baths." *Public Improvements* 1 (Sept. 15, 1899): 191–94.

———. *The Progress of the Public Bath Movement in the United States.* Paper read at First International Conference on Public and School Baths at Scheveningen, Holland, August 1912, and reprinted from *Metal Worker, Plumber and Steam Fitter* (Dec. 12, 19, 1913).

———. *Some Recent Public Rain Baths in New York City.* New York: Engineering Press, n.d.

Griscom, John H. *The Sanitary Condition of the Laboring Population of New York with Suggestions for Its Improvement.* New York: Arno Press, 1970, originally published 1845.

Hale, William H. "Personal Reminiscences of the Rev. Thomas M. Beadenkopf." *Proceedings of the American Association for Promoting Hygiene and Public Baths* (1916): 80–81.

Hooker, George C. "Mayor Quincy of Boston." *Review of Reviews* 19 (May 1899): 576–78.

Howe, Stanley H. *History, Condition and Needs of Public Baths in Manhattan.* New York Association for Improving the Condition of the Poor Publication No. 71 [1912], in Community Service Society Papers, box 37, folder 218.

## Selected Bibliography

"International Conference on Public Baths." *The Survey* 29 (Dec. 21, 1912): 351–52.

"The Janitors' Society Interested in Improved Tenements and Public Baths." *Charities* 8 (Mar. 22, 1902): 275.

*Journal of the American Association for Promoting Hygiene and Public Baths*. 1 (1918), 4–11 (1922–29).

Kelley, Robert F. G. "A Public Laundry in a Bathhouse." *American City* 26 (Jan. 1922): 43–46.

Kirkbride, Franklin B. "Philadelphia Public Baths." *Annals of the American Academy of Political and Social Science* 11 (Jan. 1898): 127–30.

———. "Private Initiative in Furnishing Public Bath Facilities." *Annals of the American Academy of Political and Social Science* 13 (March 1899): 280–84.

Koren, John. *Boston, 1822–1922, The Story of Its Government and Principal Activities During One Hundred Years*. Boston: City of Boston Printing Department, 1923.

Lee, Joseph. *Constructive and Preventive Philanthropy*. New York: Macmillan, 1902.

———. "Municipal Baths." *Charities* 6 (Mar. 2, 1901): 182–85.

Maltbie, Milo Roy. "Public Baths." *Municipal Affairs* 2 (Dec. 1898): 684–88.

Morris, Moreau. "More About the Public Rain-baths." *The Sanitarian* 37 (July 1896): 11.

New York Association for Improving the Condition of the Poor. *Communication on a System of Municipal Baths for the Borough of Manhattan, City of New York, to the Honorable Jacob A. Cantor, President of the Borough* (Feb. 25, 1902).

———. *The People's Baths*. N.d.

———. *The People's Baths: A Study on Public Baths*. Reprint from AICP Notes, No. 2, n.d.

———. *Sixteenth Annual Report, 1859* (New York: John F. Trow, 1859). *Twenty-fifth Annual Report, 1868* (New York: Trow and Smith, 1868). *Sixty-sixth Annual Report of the AICP for the year ending Sept. 30, 1909* (New York: n.p., 1909).

Paine, Ralph D. "The Bathers of the City." *Outing* 46 (Aug. 1905): 558–69.

Paton, John. *Public Baths*. 1893.

*People's Baths for Philadelphia, A Short Account of the Public Baths Association of Philadelphia, Its Organization and Objects, Charter and By-Laws*. Philadelphia: Times Printing House, 1895.

Phillips, Lily Todd. "The Branch Public Baths, Richmond, Virginia." *Journal of the American Association for Promoting Hygiene and Public Baths* 8 (1926): 47–48.

Platt, Philip S. "A Model Wet-Wash Laundry." *American City* 11 (Nov. 1914): 368–70.

Première Conférence Internationale de Bains Populaires et Scolaires tenue à Schêveningue 27–30 Août 1912 organisée par la Société Néerlandaise de Bains Populaires et Scolaires (First International Conference on People's and School Baths at Scheveningen, August 27–30, 1912, organized by the Dutch society of People's and School Baths). *Comte-rendu de Travaux*. Amsterdam: J. H. de Bussy, n.d.

Pritchard, E. R. "Free Public Baths." *World Today* 19 (Oct. 1910): 1162–63.

*Proceedings of the American Association for Promoting Hygiene and Public Baths* (1916).

Public Baths Association of Philadelphia. *Annual Reports, 1898–1904, 1907, 1912, 1928–1944.*

————. Minute Book, Scrapbooks and Papers, Library of the Historical Society of Pennsylvania.

"Public Interest in Public Baths." *Charities* 8 (Apr. 26, 1902), 382.

Quincy, Josiah. "Gymnasiums and Playgrounds." *The Sanitarian* 41 (Oct. 1898): 303–09.

————. "Municipal Progress in Boston." *Independent* 52 (Feb. 15, 1900): 424–26.

————. "Playgrounds, Baths and Gymnasia." *Journal of Social Science* 36 (Dec. 1898): 139–47.

Residents of Hull-House. *Hull House Maps and Papers.* New York: Arno Press and New York Times, 1970, originally published 1895.

Riis, Jacob A. *How the Other Half Lives: Studies Among the Tenements of New York.* N.p.: Telegraph Books, 1985, originally published 1890.

————. *The Battle with the Slum.* New York: Macmillan, 1902.

Ross, W. L. "Cleanliness and Its Advertisement, the Establishment of a Wash-House for Men in Philadelphia." *Charities* 12 (Apr. 2, 1904): 333–37.

"Simon Baruch, M.D." *Journal of the American Association for Promoting Hygiene and Public Baths* 4 (1922): 10.

Smith, Bertha H. "The Public Bath." *Outlook* 79 (Mar. 4, 1905): 566–77.

Steffens, Lincoln. *The Shame of the Cities.* New York: Hill and Wang, 1957, originally published 1904.

Stewart, Jane A. "Boston's Experience with Municipal Baths." *American Journal of Sociology* 7 (Nov. 1901): 416–22.

————. "Model Public Bath at Brookline." *American Journal of Sociology* 5 (Jan. 1900): 470–74.

Tillinghast, B. F. *Free Public Baths for Davenport.* Davenport, Ia.: Contemporary Club, 1901.

Todd, Robert E. "Four New City Baths and Gymnasiums." *The Survey* 23 (Feb. 5, 1910): 680–83.

————. "The Municipal Baths of Manhattan." *Charities* 19 (Oct. 19, 1907): 897–902.

Tolman, William Howe. *Municipal Reform Movements in the United States.* New York: Fleming H. Revell, 1895.

————. "Public Baths, or the Gospel of Cleanliness." *Yale Review* 6 (May 1897): 50–62.

————. *Social Engineering.* New York: McGraw, 1909.

————, and Hull, William I. *Handbook of Sociological Information with Especial Reference to New York City.* New York: G. P. Putnam's Sons, 1894.

# Selected Bibliography

Tucker, Frank. "Public Baths." In Robert W. Deforest and Lawrence Veiller, eds., *The Tenement House Problem,* vol. 2. New York: Macmillan, 1903, 35–55.

Veiller, Lawrence. *Housing Reform: A Handbook for Practical Use in American Cities.* New York: Charities Publication Committee, 1910.

Walker, John B. "Public Baths for the Poor." *Cosmopolitan* 9 (Aug. 1891): 414–23.

Wilcox, Delos F. *Great Cities in America.* New York: Macmillan, 1910.

Windolph, August P. "Statistical Report on Public Baths, Laundries or Wash-houses and Comfort Stations for Municipalities of 25,000 and over in the United States." *Journal of the American Association for Promoting Hygiene and Public Baths* 4 (1922): 112–15.

Wing, Frank E. "The Popularization of a Public Bath-House." *Charities* 14 (Apr. 29, 1905): 694–96.

Zueblin, Charles. *American Municipal Progress,* rev. ed. New York: Macmillan, 1916.

## Secondary Sources

Abernethy, Lloyd M. "Insurgency in Philadelphia, 1905." *Pennsylvania Magazine of History and Biography* 87 (Jan. 1963): 3–20.

———. "Progressivism, 1905–19." In Russell F. Weigley, ed., *Philadelphia: A 300-Year History.* New York: W. W. Norton, 1982, 524–65.

Abrams, Richard M. *Conservatism in a Progressive Era: Massachusetts Politics, 1900–1912.* Cambridge: Harvard University Press, 1964.

Arnold, Joseph L. "The Neighborhood and City Hall: The Origin of Neighborhood Associations in Baltimore, 1880–1911." *Journal of Urban History* 6 (Nov. 6, 1979): 3–30.

Atkins, Gordon. *Health, Housing and Poverty in New York City, 1865–1898.* Lithographed Ph.D. dissertation. Ann Arbor, Mich.: Edwards Brothers, 1947.

Baker, Paula. "The Domestication of Politics: Women and American Political Society, 1780–1920." *American Historical Review* 89 (June 1984): 620–47.

Baltzell, E. Digby. *Philadelphia Gentlemen: The Making of a National Upper Class.* Glencoe, Ill.: Free Press, 1958.

Beadenkopf, Anne. "The Baltimore Public Baths and their Founder, The Reverend Thomas M. Beadenkopf." *Maryland Historical Magazine* 45 (Sept. 1950): 201–14.

Benjamin, Philip S. "Gentlemen Reformers in the Quaker City, 1870–1912." *Political Science Quarterly* 85 (Mar. 1970): 61–79.

Blake, Nelson. *Water for the Cities.* Syracuse: Syracuse University Press, 1956.

Blodgett, Geoffrey. *The Gentle Reformers: Massachusetts Democrats in the Cleveland Era.* Cambridge: Harvard University Press, 1966.

179

———. "Yankee Leadership in a Divided City: Boston, 1860–1910." *Journal of Urban History* 8 (Aug. 1982): 371–96.

Boyer, Paul. *Urban Masses and Moral Order in America, 1820–1920.* Cambridge, Mass., and London: Harvard University Press, 1978.

Braunstein, Phillippe. "Toward Intimacy: The Fourteenth and Fifteenth Centuries." In Georges Duby, ed., *A History of Private Life,* vol. 2, *Revelations of the Medieval World,* trans. Arthur Goldhammer. Cambridge and London: Belknap Press of Harvard University, 1988, 535–630.

Bremner, Robert H. *American Philanthropy.* Chicago: University of Chicago Press, 1960.

———. *From the Depths: The Discovery of Poverty in the United States.* New York: New York University Press, 1956.

Bridenbaugh, Carl. "Baths and Watering Places of Colonial America." *William and Mary Quarterly,* 3rd ser., 3 (Apr. 1946): 151–81.

Burnham, John C. "Change in the Popularization of Health in the United States." *Bulletin of the History of Medicine* 58 (Summer 1984): 183–97.

Burns, Constance K. "The Irony of Progressive Reform: Boston, 1898–1910." In Ronald P. Formisano and Constance K. Burns, eds., *Boston, 1700–1980: The Evolution of Urban Politics.* Westport, Conn.: Greenwood Press, 1984, 133–64.

Burt, Nathaniel, and Davies, Wallace E. "The Iron Age: 1876–1905." In Russell F. Weigley, ed., *Philadelphia: A 300-Year History.* New York: W. W. Norton, 1982, 471–523.

Bushman, Richard L., and Bushman, Claudia L. "The Early History of Cleanliness in America." *Journal of American History* 74 (Mar. 1988): 1213–38.

Cavallo, Dominick. *Muscles and Morals: Organized Playgrounds and Urban Reform, 1880–1920.* Philadelphia: University of Pennyslvania Press, 1981.

Cayleff, Susan E. *Wash and Be Healed: The Water Cure Movement and Women's Health.* Philadelphia: Temple University Press, 1987.

Conway, Jill. "Women Reformers and American Culture, 1870–1930." *Journal of Social History* 5 (Winter 1971–72): 164–77.

Crooks, James B. "Maryland Progressivism." In Richard Walsh and William Lloyd Fox, eds., *Maryland: A History, 1632–1974.* Baltimore: Maryland Historical Society, 1974.

———. *Politics and Progress: The Rise of Urban Progressivism in Baltimore, 1895–1911.* Baton Rouge: Louisiana State University Press, 1968.

Davidoff, Leonore, and Hall, Catherine. *Family Fortunes: Men and Women of the English Middle Class, 1780–1850.* London: Hutchinson, 1987.

Davis, Allen F. *Spearheads for Reform: The Social Settlements and the Progressive Movement, 1890–1914.* New York: Oxford University Press, 1967.

Disbrow, Donald W. "Reform in Philadelphia Under Mayor Blankenburg, 1912–1916." *Pennsylvania History* 27 (Oct. 1960): 379–96.

# Selected Bibliography

Donegan, Jane B. *"Hydropathic Highway to Health": Women and the Water-Cure in Ante-bellum America.* Westport, Conn.: Greenwood Press, 1986.

Duffy, John. *A History of Public Health in New York City, 1866–1966.* New York: Russell Sage Foundation, 1974.

Eberlein, Harold Donaldson. "When Society First Took a Bath." *Pennsylvania Magazine of History and Biography* 67 (Jan. 1943): 30–48.

Ernst, Robert. *Immigrant Life in New York City, 1825–1863.* Port Washington, N.Y.: Ira J. Friedman, 1965.

Ford, James. *Slums and Housing,* 2 vols. Cambridge: Harvard University Press, 1936.

Fox, Bonnie R. "The Philadelphia Progressives: A Test of the Hofstadter Hays Thesis." *Pennsylvania History* 34 (Oct. 1967): 372–94.

Gettleman, Marvin E. "Philanthropy as Social Control in Late Nineteenth Century America: Some Hypotheses and Data on the Rise of Social Work." *Societas* 5 (Winter 1975): 49–59.

Gibson, Edward H., III. "Baths and Washhouses in the English Public Health Agitation, 1839–48." *Journal of the History of Medicine and Allied Sciences* 9 (Oct. 1954): 391–406.

Giedion, Siegfried. *Mechanization Takes Command.* New York: Oxford University Press, 1948.

Gitell, Marilyn, and Shtob, Teresa. "Changing Women's Roles in Political Volunteerism and Reform of the City." *Signs* 5 (Spring 1980): 567–78.

Glassberg, David. "The Design of Reform: The Public Bath Movement in America." *American Studies* 20 (Fall 1979): 5–21.

Green, Harvey. *Fit for America: Health, Fitness, Sport, and American Society.* New York: Pantheon, 1986.

Hammack, David. *Power and Society: Greater New York at the Turn of the Century.* New York: Russell Sage Foundation, 1982.

Hardy, Stephen. *How Boston Played: Sport, Recreation and Community, 1865–1915.* Boston: Northeastern University Press, 1982.

Hellebrandt, Frances A. *Simon Baruch: Introduction to the Man and His Work.* Richmond, Va.: n.p., 1950.

Holli, Melvin. *Reform in Detroit: Hazen S. Pingree and Urban Politics.* New York: Oxford University Press, 1969.

———. "Urban Reform in the Progressive Era." In Lewis L. Gould, ed. *The Progressive Era.* Syracuse: Syracuse University Press, 1974.

Hoy, Suellen M. "Municipal Housekeeping: The Role of Women in Improving Urban Sanitation Practices, 1800–1917." In Martin V. Melosi, ed., *Pollution and Reform in American Cities, 1870–1930.* Austin and London: University of Texas Press, 1980: 173–98.

Huthmacher, J. Joseph. "Charles Evans Hughes and Charles Francis Murphy: The Metamorphosis of Progressivism." *New York History* 46 (Jan. 1965): 25–40.

Keys, Thomas E., and Krusen, Frank H. "Dr. Simon Baruch and His Fight for Free Public Baths." *Archives of Physical Medicine* 26 (Sept. 1945): 549–57.

Kirschner, Don S. "The Ambiguous Legacy: Social Justice and Social Control in the Progressive Era." *Historical Reflections* 2 (Summer 1975): 69–88.

———. *The Paradox of Professionalism: Reform and Public Service in Urban America, 1900–1940*. Westport, Conn.: Greenwood Press, 1986.

Knerr, George Francis. "The Mayoral Administration of William L. Strong, New York City, 1895–97." Ph.D. dissertation, New York University, 1957.

Kramer, Howard D. "The Germ Theory and the Early Public Health Program in the United States." *Bulletin of the History of Medicine* 22 (May–June 1948): 233–47.

Kurland, Gerald. "The Amateur in Politics: The Citizen's Union Greater New York Mayoral Campaign of 1897." *New-York Historical Society Quarterly* 53 (Oct. 1969): 352–84.

Kusmer, Kenneth L. "The Functions of Organized Charity in the Progressive Era: Chicago as a Case Study." *Journal of American History* 60 (Dec. 1973): 657–78.

Ladd, Brian K. "Public Baths and Civic Improvement in Nineteenth Century German Cities." *Journal of Urban History* 14 (May 1988): 372–93.

Legan, Marshall Scott. "Hydropathy in America: A Nineteenth Century Panacea." *Bulletin of the History of Medicine* 45 (1971): 267–280.

Lubove, Roy. "The New York Association for Improving the Condition of the Poor: The Formative Years." *New-York Historical Society Quarterly* 43 (July 1959): 307–328.

———. *The Progressives and the Slums: Tenement House Reform in New York City, 1890–1917*. Pittsburgh: University of Pittsburgh Press, 1962.

McCarthy, Kathleen D. *Noblesse Oblige: Charity and Cultural Philanthropy in Chicago, 1849–1929*. Chicago: University of Chicago Press, 1982.

Mann, Arthur. *Yankee Reformers in the Urban Age*. Cambridge: Belknap Press of Harvard University, 1954.

Martin, Alfred. "On Bathing." *Ciba Symposia* 1 (Aug. 1939): 134–64.

Morantz-Sanchez, Regina Markell. *Sympathy and Science: Women Physicians in American Medicine*. New York and Oxford: Oxford University Press, 1985.

Olson, Sherry H. *Baltimore: The Building of an American City*. Baltimore: Johns Hopkins University Press, 1980.

Peterson, Jon A. "The City Beautiful Movement: Forgotten Origins and Lost Meanings." *Journal of Urban History* 2 (Aug. 1976): 415–34.

Pierce, Bessie Louise. *A History of Chicago*, vols. 1 and 3. New York: Alfred A. Knopf, 1937, 1957.

Rischin, Moses. *The Promised City: New York's Jews, 1870–1914*. New York: Harper and Row, 1970.

Rosen, George. *A History of Public Health*. New York: MD Publications, 1958.

Rosenberg, Charles E. *The Cholera Years: The United States in 1832, 1849 and 1866.* Chicago: University of Chicago Press, 1962.

Rosenkrantz, Barbara Gutmann. *Public Health and the State: Changing Views in Massachusetts, 1846–1936.* Cambridge: Harvard University Press, 1972.

Schiesl, Martin J. *The Politics of Efficiency: Municipal Administration and Reform in America, 1880–1920.* Berkeley: University of California Press, 1977.

Scott, George Ryley. *The Story of Baths and Bathing.* London: T. Werner Laurie, 1939.

Shryock, Richard H. "Sylvester Graham and the Popular Health Movement." *Mississippi Valley Historical Review* 18 (Sept. 1931): 172–83.

Sklar, Kathryn Kish. "Hull House in the 1890's: A Community of Women Reformers." *Signs* 10 (Summer 1985): 658–77.

Skolnik, Richard Stephen. "The Crystallization of Reform in New York City, 1890–1917." Ph.D. dissertation, Yale University, 1964.

Still, Bayrd. *Urban America: A History with Documents.* Boston: Little, Brown, 1974.

Swett, Steven C. "The Test of a Reformer: A Study of Seth Low." *New-York Historical Society Quarterly* 44 (Jan. 1960): 5–41.

Teaford, Jon C. *The Unheralded Triumph: City Government in America, 1870–1900.* Baltimore and London: Johns Hopkins University Press, 1984.

Thorndike, Lynn. "Sanitation, Baths, and Street-cleaning in the Middle Ages and the Renaissance." *Speculum* 3 (1928): 192–203.

Trout, Charles H. "Curley of Boston: The Search for Irish Legitimacy." In Ronald P. Formisano and Constance B. Burns, eds., *Boston, 1700–1980: The Evolution of Urban Politics.* Westport, Conn.: Greenwood Press, 1984: 165–95.

Varron, A. G. "Hygiene in the Medieval City." *Ciba Symposia* 1 (Oct. 1939): 205–14.

Ward, David. *Cities and Immigrants.* New York: Oxford University Press, 1971.

Warner, Sam Bass, Jr. *The Private City: Philadelphia in Three Periods of Its Growth.* Philadelphia: University of Pennsylvania Press, 1968.

Weiss, Harry B., and Kemble, Howard R. *The Great American Water-Cure Craze: A History of Hydropathy in the United States.* Trenton, N.J.: Past Times Press, 1967.

Whorton, James C. *Crusaders for Fitness: The History of American Health Reformers.* Princeton: Princeton University Press, 1982.

Wiebe, Robert H. *Businessmen and Reform: A Study of the Progressive Movement.* Chicago: Quadrangle Books, 1968.

Wilkie, Jacqueline S. "Submerged Sensuality: Technology and Perceptions of Bathing." *Journal of Social History* 19 (Summer 1986): 649–64.

Wilson, Margaret Gibbons. *The American Woman in Transition: The Urban Influence, 1870–1920.* Westport, Conn.: Greenwood Press, 1979.

Wortman, Marlene Stein. "Domesticating the Nineteenth-Century City." *Prospects* 3 (1977): 531–72.

Wright, Lawrence. *Clean and Decent: The Fascinating History of the Bathroom and the Water Closet.* London and Boston: Routledge and Kegan Paul, 1966.

# Index